The Sexual Wellness Handbook

Exploring Your Sexual Health, Creativity, and Pleasure

By S.S. Walker

© Copyright 2022 - All rights reserved.

The content contained within this book may not be reproduced, duplicated or transmitted without direct written permission from the author or the publisher.

Under no circumstances will any blame or legal responsibility be held against the publisher, or author, for any damages, reparation, or monetary loss due to the information contained within this book, either directly or indirectly.

Legal Notice:

This book is copyright protected. It is only for personal use. You cannot amend, distribute, sell, use, quote or paraphrase any part, or the content within this book, without the consent of the author or publisher.

Disclaimer Notice:

Please note the information contained within this document is for educational and entertainment purposes only. All effort has been executed to present accurate, up to date, reliable, complete information. No warranties of any kind are declared or implied. Readers acknowledge that the author is not engaged in the rendering of legal, financial, medical or professional advice. The content within this book has been derived from various sources. Please consult a licensed professional before attempting any techniques outlined in this book.

By reading this document, the reader agrees that under no circumstances is the author responsible for any losses, direct or indirect, that are incurred as a result of the use of the information contained within this document, including, but not limited to, errors, omissions, or inaccuracies.

Table of Contents

INTRODUCTION 8

CHAPTER 1: SEX ED 101 10
    The History of Sex Education 11

CHAPTER 2: HOW IMPORTANT IS YOUR SEXUAL WELLNESS? 15
    WHAT IS SEXUAL WELLNESS? 16
        The Importance of Maintaining Your Sexual Wellness 16

CHAPTER 3: IMPROVING YOUR SEXUAL HEALTH 22
    PHYSICAL EXAMINATIONS 22
    SEXUAL HORMONES AT DIFFERENT STAGES OF ADULTHOOD 26
    THE MOST COMMON SEXUALLY TRANSMITTED INFECTIONS 35
    IMPORTANCE OF DAILY HEALTH CARE ROUTINES 40
    PERSONAL HYGIENE ISSUES EXPERIENCED BY TRANS AND NONBINARY INDIVIDUALS 42

CHAPTER 4: EXPERIENCING SEXUAL PLEASURE 47
    ORGASMS, ONE SIZE DOES NOT FIT ALL 47

TYPES OF ORGASMS 50
    HUMAN PLEASURE TOOLS 52
    OUTERCOURSE 52
    SELF-PLEASURE 59
    FOREPLAY 61
    EXPLORING SEXUAL PLEASURE TOGETHER 64
    THE SEX POSITION BUCKET LIST 71
    GREAT SEX POSITIONS FOR A GREAT ORGASM 75

CHAPTER 5: TOOLS AND TOYS TO ELEVATE PLEASURE 83
    MOST POPULAR SEXUAL PLEASURE TOOLS 85
    EXTERNAL PLEASURE TOOLS 87
        Sex Toy Staples 88
        Dildos 88

Anal Toys *91*
Other Fun Sex Toys *94*
Sexual Aftercare *109*

CHAPTER 6: PRIORITIZING YOUR MENTAL HEALTH FOR BETTER SEX 115

Sexual Mindfulness 116
Body Positivity 118
Sex Journaling 121
Sex Therapy 123
Tantric Sex 125
Somatic Sex Education 127

CHAPTER 7: EXCITING YOUR SEXUAL CONNECTIONS 130

Dating 131
Relationships and Marriage 137
Divorce 160

CHAPTER 8: EXCITING YOUR QUEER SEXUAL CONNECTIONS 164

What Is Queer Sex? 165
Dating as a Trans Person 166
Dating Trans Women 172
Intimate Partner Violence 178
Dating a Nonbinary Person 179

CHAPTER 9: HARNESSING TECHNOLOGY FOR SEXUAL CREATIVITY 187

Technology and Sex Toys 188
Sex Podcasts 190
The Sex Tape 193

CHAPTER 10: TRENDS IN SEXUAL WELLNESS 197

CONCLUSION 201

RESOURCES 203

REFERENCES 205

Disclaimer

The information contained in this book is not intended or implied to be a substitute for professional medical advice, diagnosis, or treatment. All content, including text, images, and information contained within, is for general information purposes only.

Recognizing the Gender Spectrum

Sex and gender are not equivalent. A person's gender is an intricate and intimately interconnected relationship between social gender, body, and identity[1]. The information outlined in this book may be tailored to and varied between male, female, women, men, those with a vagina, and those with a penis. Distinctions will mostly be made based on the classifications found in the original sources that this book used for information purposes.

---

[1] "Understanding Gender," Gender Spectrum, accessed October 21, 2020. https://genderspectrum.org/articles/understanding-gender

"Sex is...perfectly natural. It's something that's pleasurable. It's enjoyable and it enhances a relationship. So why don't we learn as much as we can about it and become comfortable with ourselves as sexual human beings because we are all sexual"
—**Sue Johanson**

Introduction

"Some things are better than sex, and some are worse, but there's nothing exactly like it"

–W.C. Fields

Sex, a three-letter word that evokes a wide variety of emotions in us complicated humans. Depending on the generation, religion, or household you grew up in, our view of sex will vary from person to person.

The history of sex and the behaviors we exhibit have been surrounded by taboos, religious sanctions, and rules since the beginning of time. Sex, and the acts that accompany it, have affected cultures socially and politically around the world, dating back to prehistoric times.

Historically, men were reaping the benefits of sexual pleasure long before women ever were. We could trace this back to cavemen, but let's start at 2000 B.C.E. This is when we would first see marriage as a unit of economic trade. Men wanted to be sure they could transfer their wealth or land down to their kin, and women needed to present themselves as chaste and submissive to snag a wealthy suitor. Her only ticket to a comfortable life was her baby making oven. I can almost guarantee there was only one half of that husband and wife duo achieving climax, and it wasn't the one with the vagina.

If we were to take a peek inside the 1950s homes, what would we find? The wife in the kitchen, hair done, high-heels on and preparing dinner. The husband is relaxing in front of the television. When exactly do we think *her* last orgasm was? But I digress. She now enters the bedroom in her eleven-piece sheer ensemble, ready to please her man. The lights are off, no one will speak, missionary position, of course. After an exhausting 2.3 minutes, he will roll over and go to sleep, and she will return to the bathroom to remove her mascara and get ready for bed.

Thankfully, our mindset toward sex has changed and continues to do so. Once considered merely for procreation, it is now viewed as pleasurable, romantic, fun, and necessary. With the invention of contraceptives, a massive influx of sexual education and a positive mindset surrounding the pleasure of sex for everyone, we are finally moving forward.

In these chapters, you are going to find tips, tricks, and advice you will want to share. A brief history of sex education, improving your sexual health (or your partners), and all things pleasure. Toys, foreplay, massage, and even spanking; if it can bring you joy and orgasms, it will be in this book!

A note on the "right way to have sex". I don't think there is a right way to have sex per se. the only major requirement in a sexual experience is consent. Everything else should be up to the partners involved. We're all adults here. Not all the ideas being discussed from here on will be for everyone, that's okay. Hopefully you'll find something for you. Just keep an open mind and be ready to explore. Are you ready? Let's get started!

CHAPTER 1: Sex Ed 101

"We teach teens what we think they ought to know, and we never tell them what they want to know"
— **Sue Johanson**

The Birds and the Bees

This of course is the long since euphemism used to avoid that awkward discussion when your adorable and innocent child looks up at you and asks, "How are babies born?" It sends most parents recoiling, using excuses to discuss it later.

Parents in the past outright refused to sit across from their children and discuss intercourse, genitals, disease, pregnancy, or I dare say, *pleasure*. Roadblocks came in the form of religion, culture, and simply being uncomfortable. A mentality of, "well it worked for my parents, so it will work for me."

For generations, we sat children down and relied on nature. Feeling more comfortable describing how a bumble bee will hover over a flower, and oh, so gently, insert its stinger to obtain pollen. This is to avoid describing the actual act of a penis entering the vagina. I personally recall the birds and bees discussion as a teenager. The longer the talk went on, the more confusion enveloped my brain. Talks of sexual intercourse being how the circle of life continues. Okay, so sex is just for making babies; got it.

So, where did this "birds and bees" business even start? Many believe it began with 19th-century poet Samuel Taylor Coleridge. An excerpt from his poem, *Work Without Hope,* reads:

"All nature seems at work... the bees are stirring—birds are on the wing... and all the while, the sole unbusy thing, not honey make, nor pair, nor build, nor sing" (Coleridge, p. 1, 2021).

Over the years, different sex ed 101 lessons have emerged. The unfortunate part is there was no gradual evolution on sexuality overtime. Meaning that sex ed seems to have gone from the procreational elements right to how unsafe sex can be. We seem to have missed all the intimate, pleasurable, and fun experiences we all can enjoy. These are the items missing from the curriculum that are teaching our youth today.

The History of Sex Education

Do you recall your first sex education class? It would have been different for many of us, depending on where and when that class took place. Were you in a public, private or a religious school? Were your parents progressive enough to sit you down *before* taking the class? Regardless of the location and grade level, this was an awkward time for most of us.

If this was your first exposure to anything sex related, it could have caused more harm than good. You woke up on a random Monday, ate your breakfast, and headed off to school. You didn't know that once you sat down, you would stare up at your teacher while words like vagina, penis, and penetration would fall out of their mouth.

Pictures flashed across the screen of genitals, diseases, and body parts we had no idea we even had. Many of us left feeling confused. What if our bodies don't look like those they are showing? What are all those awful infections and diseases, and I can get those on my genitals?

As well, can you imagine for one moment, sitting through these classes aimed at educating us on all things sex, what male genitalia should entail, female genitals formed at what age. The entire time you are thinking, "my genitals don't match how I feel on the inside." No discussion on non-heterosexual sex. No discussion on gender confusion. This could lead to a confusing and isolating time for some teens.

It has taken decades to start moving the sexual education of our youth into modern times. Years of sending young adults into an already overwhelming world with out of touch and outdated information. Often times young adults are left on their own to discover their sexuality either from equally inexperienced friends or through pornography. Yah, because porn is a realistic depiction of sexual relations.

Knowledge is Pleasure

People, start taking out those mirrors and having a good look at your own bodies! If you haven't done this yet, please do. If you are wiggling in your chair at the uncomfortable thought of this, it is the mere unknown that is evoking this emotion. Get to know your bits folks.

Examine that scrotum. Magnify that vulva. If we don't know our own bodies, how are we going to tell others how to please us?

Birth Control

The world of birth control has made some advances over the years. For decades, women were offered a harsher form of hormonal pill to prevent her from having any more children. These previous generations of birth control pills would come with health risks to women, for instance:

Women who use oral contraceptives have a much greater risk of being diagnosed with cervical cancer. There was a study that found a 10% increase in the risk if you were on the pill for five years or less. The same study found that if you were taking the pill for five to nine years, your risk shot up to 60%. If you were taking oral contraceptives for ten years or more, your risk doubled (Smith, 2018).

You can imagine the relief when more options began showing themselves on the market. Currently, there are about a dozen forms of birth control available today. We now have choices of hormonal and non-hormonal types, and single use and long-term use options. As a permanent option, tubal ligation has been available for many years. This is a surgical procedure; under anesthetic, to have your fallopian tubes tied or blocked to prevent any further pregnancies. There's also a vasectomy. Again, this is a surgical procedure, and much less invasive than having a tubal ligation. There's no anesthetic needed; they snip the vas deferens tubes to keep those swimming sperms out of your semen.

The IUD, or intrauterine devices, were front and center for quite some time. A small t-shaped device, I often compare to the look of a fishing lure, is placed surgically inside the uterus. This contraption releases timely hormones into your body to prohibit conception. They last from 2 to 10 years depending on the type and manufacturer.

The Depo shot and the NuvaRing were buzz words more recently. Now made by many manufacturers, they are now more known as just "the shot", and "the ring." The shot is an injection given by your practitioner every three months. It halts your egg production, makes your cervical mucus thick and is 99% effective. Don't forget how unbelievably effective it is! The ring is flexible, and you need to insert it into your vagina each month for three weeks at a time. It also prohibits you from releasing eggs and thickens your cervical mucus. 99% effective when used correctly.

Have you heard about the patch? It is a great option as well, you can stick it anywhere on your body, just please avoid the breast areas. Leave it attached to your body for three weeks of the month, allowing it to release hormones into your body. This one too will stop your body from releasing eggs and is 99% effective when used properly.

There is a wide range of non-hormonal options. Foams, or jellies that you insert into your vagina just prior to sex, and, of course, condoms. These are less effective and can be used in conjunction with other methods.

Now that we have laid the groundwork for people to be safe while enjoying sex, let's talk about how important our sexual health and pleasure should be in our lives.

CHAPTER 2: **How Important is Your Sexual Wellness?**

"Sexuality is less about the actual act of having pretty good sex...much more about surrounding yourself with an ever-simmering sensual energy, pulsing just underneath your daily life and infusing almost everything you do"
–Sera Beak

We have all heard those catchy wellness words, haven't we? Mindfulness, self-love, peace, and well-being. We are constantly being reminded to be kind to ourselves, get the sleep we need, and nourish our bodies with healthy food choices. I want to know why we never mention sex. Why is there never a reminder to "maintain orgasms" on that list?

It is just as important as our mental and physical wellness. Social media is filled with juice diets, meditation mantras, and the joy of not giving a eff self-help books. Why is information not as readily available about sex? Why am I not scrolling through Instagram and seeing "top ten tips to achieve climax" or any sexual content that doesn't resemble pornography (not that there is anything wrong with that).

What Is Sexual Wellness?

There are a few technical definitions of sexual wellness, but basically, it is the mental, physical and emotional state when it comes to all things sex. The umbrella of sexual wellness is wide. We are talking about all things related to how you feel about your body, your sexual knowledge, and how you feel about sex.

Sexual wellness also includes your ability to have safe and pleasurable sexual experiences. Really getting to know what feels good for yourself, as well as being able to communicate that to your partner with zero shame or guilt. The ability to set boundaries in the bedroom (or wherever you choose to do the deed) and always being respectful of others' sexuality.

So, why is it so important to maintain our sexual wellness?

The Importance of Maintaining Your Sexual Wellness

We need to begin educating everyone on the importance of maintaining our sexual health. We are checking in on our physical health, and we are getting better at normalizing mental health. Fantastic, let's get this sexual health movement front and center.

Keeping our sexual wellness healthy is important. I have listed a few reasons for you to think about.

- **Keeps you healthy.** Some think sexual wellness is all about pleasure. We have to remember the benefits it brings to your health. When you equip yourself with the required knowledge regarding the benefits and risks of sexual activity, you make the best choices for your health. When we empower others with this knowledge, including unplanned pregnancy, or protection from sexually transmitted diseases, we are continuing to promote sexual wellness.

- **Enjoy a healthy sex life.** What better way to give that heart muscle a workout than knocking boots? No, seriously, a good roll in the hay gets that heart rate up and will improve your cardiovascular health. Weakened immune systems suck, okay. Before you even realize it, you are picking up every cold, flu, and virus that is around. Worse, as we age, these super viruses, and I am not naming names, can impact our health far worse than we expect. Well, guess what, getting naked and having those pleasurable orgasms helps strengthen your immune system! Yes, you heard me correctly. Now, why is this not splashed across all of those vitamin bottles and commercials for adults over twenty-five? I would much rather have multiple orgasms than take fish oil or omega-3's, but hey, maybe that's just me. So, how does it work wonders for our immune system? By releasing oxytocin, that little miracle hormone that helps fight infection. Yes, more sex and stronger immune systems, sounds like a win-win to me.

- **Improves your self-esteem.** This can be a difficult one for many. When we work on maintaining our physical health, we can be found working out, or eating better. When we are working on maintaining our mental health, we can be found visiting our therapist, or being mindful of our toxic patterns. But what about when we are maintaining our sexual wellness? This is when the tough work will come in for most. This means working on body positivity and getting comfortable in your own skin. When you are able to achieve this, it is freedom. You will start to feel more confident and sexier. This will translate into more action between the sheets. Feeling less self-conscious about your tummy, or how your partner thinks you look naked, you can focus on the pleasure. This newfound improved self-esteem will carry over into all those areas of your life where you need it most. Hold that "I just had sex" head high, you've earned it!

- **Improvement in your relationships.** I know what you are thinking. Of course, sex will improve my relationship. Well, yes, but there is more to it. Sexual wellness isn't all about the pleasure. It is heavy on the emotional intimacy side of things, too. If the sexual relationship has been stale, yes ramping up the pleasure party will check boxes in the happiness level of you both. What you may not expect is how close you both will become on all levels. Deeper conversations, long and intimate moments, that bond that only you two share. This is a trust you both have built, and having these moments opens the door for conversations about things you may want to explore in the bedroom too!

- **Sexual empowerment.** Most wouldn't expect this one, but it is important. Sexual wellness encompasses you, knowing your rights and responsibilities when it comes to sexual justice. Knowing your rights in the boudoir plays a huge role in how comfortable you will be. So, what is sexual justice? All things surrounding your right to be safe, to have pleasure, and to consent during a sexual act. Why is this important? Well, how inclined are you going to be to pull out your whip and spank your partner without any prior discussion about a safe word? Also, it can be hard to lay back and relax, allowing your partner to please you; if all that swirls around in that brain of yours is, *do they know my limits*? Nobody wants to feel awkward, hurt, unheard, or not safe. Have the discussions and empower yourself with all the knowledge you need.

There you have it, a few very important reasons why your sexual wellness matters. It is time to empower and educate yourself so that you can focus on the pleasure. This will inevitably trickle down into other areas of your life. That job won't seem so miserable. Those kids won't seem so difficult. The in-laws will seem nice as pie. So, jump on that pleasure train, only good things await.

Sexual Wellness is a Billion Dollar Industry

I am about to throw some mind-blowing statistics at you. You are going to want to sit down for this. In 2021, in the United States, the sexual wellness market (think all things sex and pleasure) was $10.3 BILLION dollars. Now that you have caught your breath, listen to this one. They are predicting that by 2029, it will climb to $17 billion (Data Bridge Market Research, 2022). Yes, you can wipe your eyes; that is not a typo.

So, I have two questions. One, where is all this money going, and two, with such a large amount of money being invested into this market, why are we not talking about it more?

Let's tackle the first question: Where is all of this money going? What has spiked this market and the projections?

The number one item to drive this number up is condoms. Yes, that tiny, slippery, little bugger is a billion dollar hot ticket item. Now, condoms have come a very long way since their inception. The first condom was invented in 1855, by none other than Charles Goodyear. Yes, the tire guy! These first condoms were the same thickness of a bicycle tire and you had to be custom fitted for one (Team, 2020). Doesn't that sound delightful? Decades have passed, and now we have a much more convenient and inexpensive birth control method. Condoms also help stop the spread of sexually transmitted infections or STIs and diseases.

We have also come leaps and bounds in educating our communities on the importance of using condoms. Better sex education in our schools has boosted sales on condoms. And most of us have seen the readily available baskets of free condoms in health clinics and some colleges and high schools.

So these are the main drivers that have caused condom sales to explode, but we also know they don't count for all of the increased sales in the sexual wellness market. So, where is all that other money coming from? There coming from sex toys, erotic lingerie, sexual body wash, pregnancy tests, performance enhancers, lubricants, contraceptives, and antifungal agents.

These are how we're spending our well-earned money in the sexual wellness industry. It's important to start normalizing the sexual wellness market. Normalize using lubricants for vaginal dryness and because it feels so fantastic. Normalize wearing that leather catsuit while asking to be spanked. And normalize owning sex toys. Why? Because sexual pleasure contributes to our greater holistic wellness...(and orgasms are great).

CHAPTER 3: Improving Your Sexual Health

"Some of the best moments in life are the ones you can't tell anyone about"
–**Anonymous**

I've made mention on the importance of maintaining your sexual wellness and discussed the need to see our doctor for our physical health, and our therapist for our mental health. But we also need to direct our attention to our sexual health in particular.

Physical Examinations

When was the last time you visited your physician regarding your naughty bits? Yep, you know what I am talking about, draped in the paper dress, feet in the stirrups making small talk while they do whatever it is they do down below. There is an entire slew of exams you should be having annually to keep your sexual health in perfect shape. I know you are booking those dentist appointments and eye exams, so there should be no excuse to add this appointment either. Keep those vaginas, breasts, and penises in tip-top shape! What exams should you be scheduling? So glad you asked; I have listed them out for you.

- **A physical exam:** This should include a conversation about any changes you have seen throughout the year. Be prepared to discuss whether there has been any changes in your general health, job, relationship, medications, sleep and eating patterns. Get your vitals checked, and of course blood work. But these are the basics.

The remainder of the tests below are based on either the known medical test for a specific body part or medical screenings. Please pay keen attention to any that may apply to your body.

- **Abdominal Aortic Aneurysm screening:** heart disease is the number one killer for men, so it is not surprising that this test is so important. It is a screening done once, and an easy test done by ultrasound. It is recommended around the age of 60 for those who have a history of smoking.

- **Breast exam:** yes, it can be awkward having your doctor squeezing your boobs, but these are an absolute must. Do yourself a favor and have your doctor show you how to conduct these tests on yourself. Regular self-exams can save your life.

- **Cholesterol test:** depending on your health history consider starting regular cholesterol checks by the age of 45. If you have a family history of heart disease or diabetes, you should begin cholesterol checks by age 20.

- **Mammogram:** the breast examination test. This test saves lives every day. Breast cancer is the most common cancer among women. It is estimated that, in 2022, 28,600 Canadian women will be diagnosed with breast cancer, and 5,500 will die from it (Lee, 2020). This disease should be a part of your sexual health discussions. In those of us with a lower risk for breast cancer, a mammogram is recommended every two years. You will typically start having them at age 50. If you have a family history of breast cancer, your mammograms will start earlier.

- **Osteoporosis screening:** Well, that took a quick turn, didn't it? It is inevitable that as we age, things like bone density become important. Scans for your bone density will start happening around age 60. If you are someone who suffers from autoimmune diseases, you may have these sooner.

- **Pap smear:** this is a screening primarily for cervical cancer. Do not skip out on it. No, it is not pleasant, but it could save your life. Legs up in the stirrups while you make small talk with the doctor. A super long cotton swab is inserted into your vagina and then it is sent off for analysis. You should begin this test no later than age 21, but usually once you become sexually active. Once the first one is complete, screenings are conducted every two years or so. Depending on your physician, and where you live, your screenings may change to once every five years after the age of 40. Once you hit the age of 65, you most likely will no longer require the stirrup greeting, as I like to call it.

- **Pelvic exam:** it should be a regular part of your physical exam to have your pelvic area examined. Your physician is visually examining your genitals for signs of STIs, and well as feeling inside for any growths or abnormalities. Sounds wonderful right? Just remind yourself that a healthy body and healthy genitalia means continued healthy sex and pleasure.

- **Prostate cancer screening:** the exam for your prostate. Your physician, all gloved up, will place a finger or two, into your rectal cavity, in search of your prostate. They are checking to be sure it is not swollen. Screening typically begins at age 50, but again, if a strong family history presents itself, you could be starting at age 40. As I mentioned previously, do not skip this exam. Is it awkward and slightly embarrassing to some? Sure, but it can save lives.

- **Testicular exam:** this is a very common assessment to have the physician check your testicles for any abnormalities. They will be looking for odd lumps, bumps, or tenderness. Be sure to mention anything out of the ordinary that you may have noticed as well.

Sexual Hormones at Different Stages of Adulthood

As a teenager, hormones caused us to have those terrible breakouts on our faces and become upset for reasons we didn't understand. But what is a hormone, anyway? A hormone is actually a naturally occurring substance in your body. They are the neat little things that translate messages between organs and cells. Every human on this planet carries male and female hormones. That is your science lesson for today; you are welcome. As adults, how do our sex hormones affect us, and how do they change throughout our adult life? The journey for all sexes is very different.

Hormonal Changes in Women

In women, the two sex hormones are progesterone and estrogen. Most are aware that testosterone is a male hormone, but women produce this too and need a small amount to stay balanced.

Estrogen
Considered the queen of the female hormones, most of it comes from the ovaries. A teeny tiny amount is secreted from the fat cells and adrenal glands. Estrogen is the mother ship when it comes to sexual development and reproduction. Without estrogen, you would not have puberty, menstruation, pregnancy or menopause.

Progesterone

This is the sex hormone that is produced only after ovulation. Women, when pregnant, will have the added bonus of a placenta that produces it as well. Progesterone has a significant job. It has the responsibility of preparing the lining of the uterus for when that egg is ready to be fertilized. We also need this miracle sex hormone to help support a pregnancy; without it, carrying a baby to term would not be possible. Progesterone also has the abilities to cease the production of estrogen after ovulation.

Hormonal Changes throughout a Woman's Life

Women's bodies change significantly from childhood, through puberty, and into adulthood. As our bodies change, our hormonal needs do as well. As we travel through our hormonal journey, we begin to see how our fluctuating hormonal levels can affect us differently.

All three hormones, estrogen, progesterone, and testosterone are key factors in female sexual libido, as well as how women function, sexually. Hormone testing has shown that women are at their sexual peak just before ovulation and that libido often fluctuates less after menopause.

Childbirth can wreak havoc on hormone levels. After childbirth, all your levels begin to nosedive. Don't panic too much, they are just trying to reach their pre-pregnancy levels. Studies are now showing, though, that this drastic, sudden drop in hormone levels could be a contributing factor in postpartum depression (Healthline, 2018).

Perimenopause is the time before menopause when hormone levels start to plummet. As this happens, one of the first things you may notice is a dry vagina. Yep, vaginal moisture begins to dry up like the Sahara Desert. No wonder why libido begins to take a dive. I truly hope this is the time you begin experimenting with lube if you haven't already. It is a game changer, trust me.

You're considered to be in menopause once you have missed twelve periods. No more menstruation, no more buying period products, and no more premenstrual syndrome. But, those rapidly plunging hormone levels mean an increased risk for osteoporosis, heart disease, and chin hair. Make nice with your esthetician; they will become like family.

Hormonal Changes in Men

As indicated above, it is easy to see how often women's hormone levels are disrupted. Puberty, pregnancy, and menopause all affect those levels. With men, it is a different story. Obviously, you don't have those same instances disturbing those levels. Because of this, you have a much more gradual decline in testosterone over the years.

Testosterone production begins in puberty. This continues and slowly increases, reaching its max around the age of 30. Men have a solid ten years of steady hormone levels, before starting to decline, around age 40. This is when your testosterone levels begin to slowly drop off. You may start to panic when you hear this statistic, but it only declines around 1% each year. It will stay this way until age 75, when that jumps to 3% (Roser et al., 2013).

For men, there is some great news. There are some solid ways that you can slow this process down. I have listed them below.

- **Keep an eye on your body weight.** A higher body mass index or BMI and an increase in body fat can be tied to a more rapid decline in testosterone. Keeping up on a healthy balanced diet and moderate exercise can help slow that hormone level drop.

- **Prevent getting type 2 diabetes or hypertension**. Again, keep an eye on your diet and exercise. These two things combined are what will keep you from getting type 2 diabetes.

- **Don't smoke**. It causes a much faster decline in those testosterone levels. It's dangerous for your health and those around you. Smoking causes cancer, yellow teeth and bad breath.

- **Psychological factors.** Psychological factors can have an impact on how quickly testosterone levels drop. Those with chronic stress, depression, or bad sleep habits experienced a faster rate of decline.

Hormones in the Nonbinary/Trans Community

Forty-three percent of millennials reported knowing someone who uses gender neutral pronouns and that number increases to 56% of Gen-Z. In the most recent and largest survey of transgender individuals in the United States, 35% said they identified as non-binary (Ford et al., 2016).The need to include greater attention to the medical and mental health concerns of genderqueer people in our health care system is critical.

Transgender individuals have come to use hormone therapy as an integral part of their transitioning process. Many have also used gender-affirming hormone therapy or GAHT to manage gender dysphoria. This is most often used for those transitioning from masculine to feminine but overtime there has been a greater need for hormone therapy.

Microdosing

Microdosing hormones is known as a low-dose form of gender-affirming hormone therapy. Doing this allows those who identify as nonbinary to acquire subtle changes in their body. For instance, by taking estrogen for gender feminization, you will increase breast growth, increase the softness of your skin, and reduce the hair growth on both the body and face. By ingesting testosterone on the other hand, you will notice gender masculinization in the form of body and facial hair, more muscle mass in targeted areas, and a deeper voice.

It's next to impossible to find doctors that will support low-dose GAHT because hormone therapy is an all-or-nothing practice in the U.S. healthcare system (Proschan, 2021). You either want to do everything, or nothing. They cannot see a middle ground here.

Unfortunately, the mental benefits of GAHT are not as openly discussed as the physical, given the closeness of this treatment to gender-affirming surgeries. We have to be mindful of the fact that, for many non-cisgender people, hormones work wonders for inner anxiety, depression, and the extreme frustration that constitutes gender dysphoria. Transitioning or exploring the gender binary is vastly different for each and every person.

Hormones can be part of this journey, but they shouldn't dictate how "manly" or "womanly" a person is. Now, with an increased accessibility to hormones, and more transgender and nonbinary supportive providers, the ability to try GAHT is more accessible than before.

Common Health Problems That Affect Sexual Health and What to do About Them

Each of us experiences stress and the mundane routine of everyday living. Dropping the kids at school, getting to work, making dinner, doing the laundry, sleeping, and repeating. It leaves very little room for sex or pleasure. A quick fix for this is intentionally setting aside time. Time for quiet and relaxation; time to breathe and regulate our emotions. You will be amazed at how quickly you will become attuned with your wants, needs, and desires. When you quiet the chaos, you can hear your own wishes.

I have listed what would be the most common health problems that could get in the way of your sexual health, and what you can do about them.

- **Stress:** This is a big one in most people's lives. It can not only affect your sex life, but it can end relationships if not dealt with. Communication is key here, so instead of closing up, talk it out. If you don't feel you can talk openly with your partner yet, talk to a therapist. Find an outlet, whether that is smashing golf balls, or blowing off steam at the gym. Stress is only an issue when it doesn't have an outlet.

- **Diabetes:** When we think of diabetes we think of insulin resistance, too much sugar, and maybe diabetic comas. Did you know that diabetic neuropathy is a form of nerve damage, and it can also affect the genitals. In fact, it can cause you to have no feeling in your naughty bits. It can lead to erectile dysfunction, or the inability to orgasm. Working closely with a nutritionist to get your diet in check can drastically increase your chances of reversing your type 2 diabetes.

- **Sleep apnea:** 60% of men with sleep apnea have a decreased sex drive. It is thought that the severe lack of sleep is the contributing factor. In fact, when one partner isn't getting a sound sleep due to sleep apnea, there is a great chance the other isn't either. With both constantly being exhausted, sex is often left on the back burner. Book a sleep study test and get yourself one of the CPAP machines. Save your relationship, your sex life AND get that sleep you've been missing for years.

- **Obesity:** You may face difficulties being adventurous with sex positions. Being overweight actually narrows the blood vessels that travel to your genitals. What does this mean for sex? Well, it actually makes it much more difficult to reach climax. So listen, nobody needs that kind of pressure. Getting into an exercise and healthy eating routine is going to make you feel amazing, and once those orgasms start, you will feel like a champion.

- **Hormonal imbalance:** As we discussed earlier, once your hormones start jumping all over the place during childbirth, breastfeeding, or menopause, your body changes a lot. From vaginal dryness, to a dried-up libido, you don't know where to turn. Do yourself a favor and explore that lube aisle. Nobody wants to entertain the idea of inserting anything into their vagina when they know it will be painful. If your mood swings and night sweats are more than you, or your partner can handle, talk to your doctor and see if they can offer you any relief. Speak with your nutritionist or holistic team, as they will all have wonderful ideas as well.

- **Vaginal dryness:** This is a reality for many women. It is nothing to be ashamed about, it happens to many women. Clearly, I am a huge fan of lube. I started using it way before it was necessary. Start exploring with it on your own. See which ones you enjoy, flavored, scented, smooth, or even heated...have fun and enjoy.

- **Yeast infections:** Before we get started on this one, I want to reassure you just how common they are. Over one million women, each year, contract a yeast infection in the United States. It is a fungal infection caused by the yeast candida, which is always present in your body, but when it decides to grow on the outside, you have a yeast infection. These are just miserable and make us feel miserable. In case you were wondering, no, you should not have sex if you have a yeast infection, they are highly contagious. They can be painful, itchy, and can cause burning. In some instances you may need a prescription to clear the infection. For future preventative measures, you can wear cotton underwear, as they allow more air flow around your vagina. You should not be douching, as it disturbs the normal pH level of your vagina, and always practice good hygiene.

- **Bacterial vaginosis:** The hub of vaginal bacterial growth. This one is most associated with odor and discharge. It is persistent and can stay with vagina owners for great lengths of time. A direct result of lack of vaginal acidity, sexual activity, inserting sex toys that are not cleaned properly, unprotected sex, or frequent douching. To remedy this one, seeing your doctor immediately for an antibiotic and maintaining impeccable hygiene will get you on the road to recovery.

- **Erectile dysfunction:** This one can be caused by physical or psychological issues, which is what makes it a tricky beast. Sleep apnea can cause penises some issues. The lack of oxygen to the organ plays into it. Regardless, you need to speak to your doctor if this issue becomes regular. It can be a sign of heart issues or high blood pressure. Have no fear; there are some great medications or therapies that can help.

The Most Common Sexually Transmitted Infections

Sexually transmitted infections or STIs have been a part of society for generations. With the advancements in today's society, you should be taking the necessary precautions to protect yourself. I have compiled a list of the eight most common STIs and their statistics.

- **Human Papillomavirus (HPV)**

    The human papillomavirus is a fairly newer STI, made very public mostly because of the vaccine blitz to our youth about ten years ago. The Center for Disease Control or CDC states that an approximate 43 million cases of HPV were reported in 2018, with most of those in their teens and 20s (Center for Disease Control and Prevention, 2021). A large portion of HPV types will cause genital warts. The most cause for concern is the strains of this virus that can cause cervical cancer, cancer of the mouth, throat, or penis. HPV is detected through a routine pap smear, so do not skip these for your own sake and that of your partner. If you are not yet vaccinated, getting that will drastically reduce your risk from the strains causing cancer. To protect yourself from HPV, consider getting vaccinated. As a back-up, use those condoms each and every time you engage in sexual activity.

- **Herpes**

  Herpes is one of the most expensive, and contagious STIs. It has been estimated that for suppressive therapy, the average cost is $240 to $2,580 annually. That is one very expensive unprotected sexual experience. Herpes consists of two viral strains: *herpes simplex type 1 (HSV-1)* and *herpes simplex type 2 (HSV-2)*. If you contract oral herpes, you may notice fever blisters or the dreaded cold sore. I can't forget to mention anal and genital sores as well. Herpes can also affect fetuses, so you must inform your doctor if you think you might be pregnant. To protect yourself from herpes, you should be using condoms faithfully, be monogamous or limit the number of sexual partners you have.

- **Syphilis**

  A 2022 sexually transmitted disease study indicates that sexual activity, homelessness, an HIV diagnosis, as well as a history of tobacco or drug use as risk factors for syphilis, which is caused by a bacterium called treponema pallidum (Ford et al., 2022). Transmissible by touching a syphilis sore, infection can begin with a hard, painless sore on the mouth, penis, anus, or vagina. Often, these sores go unnoticed because they don't cause any discomfort. Unfortunately, the infection will progress and if left untreated, it can damage the liver, heart, bones, joints and skin. To protect yourself from syphilis, abstain from sex with someone who has the infection, use a condom and don't share needles.

- **Hepatitis**

    Hepatitis can be transmitted sexually and can cause a variety of symptoms. It shows itself in varying forms: fatigue, dark urine, vomiting, stomach pain, and yellowing of the skin and eyes. Occasionally sexually transmitted, Hepatitis A virus (HAV) is found in feces. It will often spread throughout an entire family because of close contact. Hepatitis B virus (HBV) is sexually transmissible. Infection can also be transmitted by sharing needles and passed from mother to child during delivery. A vaccine for Hepatitis A and B is available. To prevent hepatitis from coming into your life, consider getting vaccinated. Use those condoms and don't share needles. If you know your partner is infected, keep your personal toiletry items separate.

- **Trichomoniasis**

    This one is not like the rest of the STIs on the list. It is, in fact, a parasite infection. Though it is one of the most curable STIs, it can cause severe symptoms when it comes to pregnant women. According to a 2021 International Journal of Obstetrics and Gynecology review, this parasitic infection can result in early delivery, low birthweight, and pre-labor rupture of membranes. Symptoms of trichomoniasis look like a very angry vagina. Burning, redness, a whole bunch of itching and soreness. You will find discomfort when you pee and notice a discharge with an odor. Irritation on the inside of the penis and burning when you pee are also notable symptoms. In many cases, penis owners won't have any symptoms and may spread this STI to their partners. To prevent yourself from contracting trichomoniasis, get those condoms out and use them without fail every time you engage in sex. Don't forget oral sex, use those condoms, or dental dams to protect yourself here too.

- **Gonorrhea**

  Gonorrhea seems to be making a comeback since the pandemic. The CDC is also informing us that there is a brand new antibiotic-resistant brew surfacing, making it hard to treat while it continues to spread. This STI thrives in all warm and moist areas like your eyes, anus, vagina, and throat. The most common signs are genital discharge and pain or burning when you pee. If you have a vagina and suspect you may have gonorrhea, don't let it go untreated. You could find yourself with pelvic inflammatory disease. To prevent gonorrhea, practice abstinence, or commit to a long-term relationship with someone who is willing to be tested before you engage in sexual activity.

- **Chlamydia**

  The bacterium chlamydia trachomatis is responsible for what makes up this STI, which often goes undetected due to lack of symptoms. Some do experience abnormal penile or vaginal discharge. Much like gonorrhea, chlamydia has the potential to result in pelvic inflammatory disease (PID) in women. This can result in infertility or even ectopic pregnancy. The U.S. Preventive Services Task Force updated its guidance on chlamydia in 2021. According to the new guidelines, all sexually active women ages 24 and younger should be screened (Davidson et al., 2021). The best way to protect yourself from chlamydia is condoms, during sex, and over the genitals, during oral sex. Also, be mindful of sharing sex toys, keeping them clean, or using condoms over them as well.

- **Human Immunodeficiency Virus (HIV)**

There have been amazing new developments that are good news, because the implications for HIV are serious. HIV has the potential to lead to AIDS—the acquired immune deficiency syndrome. This STI attacks and weakens the immune system. The CDC claims that among new cases of HIV in 2019, 65% came from male-to-male direct sexual contact (CDC, 2019). Another 23% came from heterosexual contact, while 7% came from injection drug use. If you have an early-stage of HIV, you can experience fever, headache, sore muscles, swollen glands, muscle aches, or extreme fatigue. If treated, the viral load can disappear for years. The best way to protect yourself from HIV is abstinence, not sharing needles, and using condoms each and every time you engage in sexual activity.

Importance of Daily Health Care Routines

While we are discussing all of the reasons, we may be turned on or off in the bedroom, we should touch on "maintenance." Those things you should be doing routinely to keep things neat, trim, and tidy so you feel your absolute best. We all know that when you feel your best, you do your best!

Clean Intimate Care
What does it look like when you step into your shower? Is there one bottle of body wash and multiple bottles of shampoo? Do you still prefer bar soap? Do you mix up the scents or have you been using the same one since high school? How much time and consideration do you give to the products you use to clean your genitals? Who taught you the proper way to clean your bits? Trust me, there are many complicated places down there, and if you were never given proper instruction, you may just be lathering, rinsing, and hoping for the best.

In all honesty, you shouldn't be using any of those harsh body washes or soaps on your genitals, ever...

Your vulva, especially, will get angry, red, and itchy if you attempt to use those chemicals. This is your vagina's way of reminding you that it already has its own balanced pH cleaning system. Nothing more is required than a very mild soap and warm water on the outside of the vagina. Or even just water. It's like a self-cleaning oven.

Similarly, if you have a penis, don't overdue the chemicals, and be sure to use unscented soap on your bits too. If you are uncircumcised, be sure you are getting into all those cracks and crevices so you can proudly present your penis. Your goal here is to keep all the parts clean daily including your armpits, breasts, butt and so on.

Grooming Routines

Not everyone cares to groom themselves. To each is own and as long as you are confident in your body, so be it. However for those who like to keep your nether regions tidy, below are some grooming routines you'll need to be maintaining regardless of the parts you have. Let's start from top to bottom.

- **Head and Hair**. Whether you are rocking those luscious locks or shaving it smooth, hair maintenance is at the top. There is no need to be washing your hair every day, you are just stripping all those natural oils out. Every 2-3 days is perfect. Pick a scent that is for you. Gone are the days when we had to smell like roses or gunpowder.

- **Armpits**. No foul odor ever! This is non-negotiable. If you choose to shave, wax, sugar, or let your flow grow, just keep it clean. Your deodorant game should be unique to you as well.

- **Breasts.** If you were born with them, bought them, or grew them, breasts are a big responsibility. Used for feeding humans, entertaining humans, and even ourselves. Keeping your breasts clean and healthy is a priority. Keep those tah-tahs clean and healthy!

- **Genitals.** Regardless of what you are packing, for the love of all things horny, keep it clean. Sweat, bodily fluids (our own or others) and anything else that finds its way there needs to be cleaned or we can end up with infections. Can I just say here that not only can this be serious, but it is so uncomfortable. Nip this in the bud and clean, clean, clean! Harsh scents and chemicals are not for the genitals people. This too will provide hours of irritation.

- **Body hair.** It is everywhere, and it can be glorious or hide odor. If you choose to keep it, clean it. If you choose to rid yourself of it, moisturize that freshly shaven skin, you will thank yourself later.

Remember, with all of these grooming tips, you are what matters. Scents, materials, approaches, all depend on what makes you feel beautiful, empowered and sexy!

Personal Hygiene Issues Experienced by Trans and Nonbinary Individuals

A 2021 study by the Williams Institute, showed approximately 1.2 million Americans (or 11% of the LGBTQ2S++ population) identify as nonbinary or trans. This study showed that 94% of nonbinary adults have considered suicide at some point in their lives (Srikanth, 2021).

These adults face additional stress that is typically caused by psychological stress. Researchers claim this can be from things like, poor, uninformed, and discriminatory treatment from healthcare, to basic challenges in personal hygiene (O'Mann, 2021). "Being trans/nonbinary is a unique kind of gender minority experience because you are constantly surrounded by binary-identified people," said study author, Bianca Wilson. Discrimination can affect your daily hygiene routines on so many levels, so what can we do to be more aware and sensitive about them?

Gender Dysphoria and Menstruation

Gender dysphoria individuals feel a disconnect between gender identity and their actual gender assigned sex at birth. Keep in mind that nonbinary and transgender people can have gender dysphoria as well. This is typically triggered when a part of their body feels foreign or that it just doesn't belong. This tends to peak around menstruation.

As stated in research by Sarah E. Frank, "Menstruation has been historically known as a function of the female body that affects women. Trans and nonbinary people face this biological function as a potential social signal of gender/sex identity."

These are specific and tend to be embarrassing challenges. Menstruation and personal hygiene have always presented challenges for all of us, but throw in these additional challenges and they create anxiety and stress. Imagine being in a men's bathroom stall, changing your maxi pad, only to discover they don't tend to keep trash bins there. Or, again, you are precariously perched over the toilet, taking care of your period business, when other men enter that bathroom. We all know that opening a pad sounds as though you are smashing glass or opening Christmas presents. The echo alone can make one cringe. All these sounds are unfamiliar in a men's bathroom. (Frank, 2020).

Making Improvements

It is evident that we need more education and empowerment in these areas. We are making strides and advancements, but we need to do more. We want everyone to feel comfortable in their bodies. We need this comfort level in order to be encouraged to stay on top of our exams. They can save our lives.

Some small advances in the area of menstrual hygiene have begun. The launch of trans and nonbinary-friendly menstruation companies like THINX (which makes boy shorts/briefs for menstruation that empower trans men). This company keeps comfort, discreteness and fashion in mind. They come in many types, and the absorbency lasts for almost a full day. You can imagine what a difference it can make simply changing out of these in a public bathroom.

We know that more needs to be done. Beginning by educating all of the menstrual companies. Let's start marketing with less over the top stereotypically feminine designs and colors and stick to the more gender-neutral tones. I don't want to speak for all humans out here, but even as a young teen, I was always mortified to have to put that hot pink box up on the pharmacy counter.

Something as simple as placing trash cans in all washrooms. Most people would find it convenient to have a bin in their stall and not even question its presence. This is a small solution that can make it a little less obvious when using your sanitary products.

When it comes to healthcare, this is a mountain that we continue to climb. Continued education and understanding is key here. As we discussed earlier, routine medical exams are important for your sexual health. As a trans or non-binary individual, there are going to be times that you have to advocate for your health more ardently than those who are not. If it brings you comfort and support, take in reinforcements. When the day comes for an exam, take your strongest advocate. Make it clear to the healthcare team what you are comfortable with and what you are not. It is okay to take the time you need to build a trust level with your medical team first. This is your body, your vessel, so you steer the boat.

Gender-Affirming Hygiene Products
Hygiene products such as lotions, shampoos, and deodorants are often marketed in stereotypical colors and masculine or feminine fragrances. You usually walk down the aisle, women's choice on one side, men on the other. A straight divide down the middle. This can be stressful and cause anxiety for nonbinary people. There is a growing number of companies making a solid attempt to rid the world of gender stereotypes in personal hygiene products. The big contenders on the market right now to watch for are Noto (which presents a fluid, non-conformist vision of

beauty for the face and body), Ursa Major (which believes that 'skin is skin' and caters to the needs of different types of skin), and State of Menopause (O'Mann, 2021).

Tips For Reducing Triggers

Attempting to reduce triggers can go a long way for nonbinary/trans people when it comes to personal hygiene. For example, if having showers causes anxiety, consider low lighting and soft music. If excessive body hair is an issue, consider trusting a friend to help with waxing those areas you can't reach. For those personal hygiene tasks, you know have to be tackled but bring you nothing but angst, consider pleasant distractions such as pets, your favorite music, or bingeing Netflix to take you to a happy place (Vered Counseling, 2019).

Regular Maintenance

As we wrap up this chapter, I just want to remind you of the regular maintenance you should be upkeeping. It is those small things that you can do every day to keep yourself on track to feeling great physically, mentally and sexually.

Keep working towards improved sleep habits. Strive for regular exercise, better eating habits, and drinking that water daily. It is also very important that you keep in touch with your doctor on a regular basis to keep on top of those tests and screenings we discussed.

Okay, we need to move on to the next chapter because I can't wait another minute to discuss all things pleasure!

CHAPTER 4: Experiencing Sexual Pleasure

"I don't have a dirty mind, I have a sexy imagination"—**Unknown**

Many say that most people are influenced by pleasure and pain. I can't say they're wrong. For me, experiencing sexual pleasure has been one of the best parts of adulthood. Sexual pleasure adds much more richness to our lives than any other activity. However, depending on your experiences and who you've experienced them with, our level of pleasure can vary greatly. In the next two chapters, I want to spend time discussing the myriad of ways to achieve pleasure both alone and together, and as giver and receiver.

Orgasms, One Size Does Not Fit All

The big "O" is the pinnacle of sex, or so the picture has been painted for us. The orgasm has had the buildup (pun intended) for so long, nobody can confirm when all the hoopla started. Focus on the goal, the endgame, the finish line, and the journey never mattered. It has taken years of research and strong voices to inform people that not everyone orgasms from penetration, and if you didn't know that before reading this, you have purchased the perfect book. Orgasms come in so many different variations, and educating yourself on this will only increase your own pleasure and what you offer your partners.

So, what is an orgasm? The American Psychological Association (APA) defines it as "When a person is able to reach peak pleasure, then the body relaxes, then releases tension, the perineal muscles, anal sphincter, and reproductive organs rhythmically contract" (McIntosh, 2018, para.4).

Typically with a penile orgasm, it is evident from your ejaculation. For clitoral ones, it is a different story. The vaginal walls release and contract, often quickly. You too have the ability to orgasm, when the moons align, and everyone knows their role!

Way back in 1966, there were two researchers, William Master and Virginia Johnson who came up with a four-phase model of orgasms: excitement, plateau, orgasm, and resolution (Rowland & Gutierrez, 2017).

Not long after, another researcher by the name of Dr. Helen Kaplan introduced another model. Hers differed from the earlier model as she believed desire was important to achieve orgasm. Her model included desire, excitement, and orgasm (Rowland & Gutierrez, 2017).

What Happens During an Orgasm?

No two orgasms are created equal; I believe that would make a great t-shirt. Honestly, it is true. The intention is to feel pleasure. You should feel mind-numbing, toe-curling, eyes rolling into the back of your head, pleasure in your genitals, but it does resonate through most of your body. It is also quite normal for you to feel extremely relaxed and a bit sleepy afterwards. So, for all of those out there who give your partner grief for dozing off after sex, orgasms are exhausting!

As I mentioned, we don't all experience orgasms the same way. For clitoral orgasms, you will feel a tightening in both your anus and your vagina. Ready for another interesting fact? Both of these areas will contract at a rate of one every single second, about a dozen times (McIntosh, 2018). It's okay if you're sitting there thinking, *that does not happen to me.* Not all clitoral orgasms are experienced like this. If you do, congratulations. A large percentage of people will report a very sensitive clitoris after orgasm though. For the penile orgasm, they too will have contracting muscles in the anus and the penis, but typically just once or twice as they ejaculate. How much does the penis ejaculate? It's usually one to two tablespoons at the most. The head of the penis is super sensitive after orgasm, to the point it may feel uncomfortable to the touch.

Orgasms Are Healthy

Yes, you read that right. There are legitimate health benefits to having those amazing and pleasurable orgasms.

Frontiers in Public Health conducted a thorough study of sex and sleep. They wanted to dig deeper into the ideation of orgasms and better sleep patterns. The study consisted of 442 females and 336 males, with an average age of 35. When they finished the study, they found that orgasms with a partner showed improved overall sleep patterns. When they looked at orgasms brought on through self-pleasure, not only was there an improvement in overall sleep, but it took much less time to actually fall asleep (Lastella et al., 2019).

I wish I could announce these findings to all the insomniacs of the world. Ditch the sleeping pills and get a few great sex toys, it's a win-win.

So, what other health benefits can we achieve through more orgasms? We know from earlier in the book that we are flooded with that feel good hormone, oxytocin after orgasm, and it does all kinds of wonderful things for us. One of the big ones is reducing our chance of ovarian cancer. It also helps lower our anxiety levels, and we can all do with a little of that. There has been a recent study regarding prostate cancer. It has been shown that men who ejaculate more often may reduce their chances of getting this type of cancer. Doctors have been diagnosing these men less often (Rider et al., 2016).

Types of Orgasms

In the land of pleasure and sex, were you aware there were more than one kind of orgasm? Hold on tight as we break down these for you and open up a world for you to explore.

- **Nipple orgasms:** Yes, it is true, an orgasm can be reached through the licking, sucking, tucking, and any other form of stimulation you can imagine. If you have been ignoring this erogenous zone, you may want to rethink it.

- **G-spot orgasms:** The ever-elusive G-spot. Once you master locating it, this orgasm is one you won't soon forget. Get researching and read the section we have included in this book. You won't regret it.

- **Anal orgasm:** It has been said that there are some folks who enjoy the lip biting orgasm during anal sex. I will call them lucky.

- **Blended orgasm:** This is one of the most glorious orgasms to achieve, a combination of both a vaginal and a clitoral orgasm simultaneously.

- **Clitoral orgasm:** The be all and end all. This orgasm is fulfilled by tickling that button, a.k.a. the clitoris. The majority of vagina owners orgasm this way.

- **Vaginal orgasm:** Penetration is the name of the game here. Most would assume that is how orgasm is achieved here, but oftentimes, it is the rubbing against the clitoris that does the trick.

- **Multiple orgasm:** I saved the best for last. A superhero… okay, just a normal human, who can achieve orgasms in quick succession of each other. Clitoral orgasms in general don't need much recovery time between, so this is usually reserved for them. Granted, there are superhero erection havers capable of achieving this as well.

There you have it; the wonderful world of orgasms. May you be blessed with many!

Human Pleasure Tools

A good place to begin is with you. You are in need of a release, pleasure, happiness, joy, whatever you need, and you are all you have. You are the human tool. First up on our list is outercourse.

Outercourse

There are always two questions surrounding the topic of outercourse: What is it, and is it the same as abstinence? Both are great questions, so let's explore this topic a bit more.

What is Outercourse?

Most get the basic gist of outercourse just by the name. Outer versus intercourse would give an indication that we may be talking about any and all sexual activity without penetration. However, this leaves us open to debate.

While penetration can mean penis entering the vagina or anus to some, for others, it could mean using fingers or tongue, or sex toys. At the same time, some people have a strict preference to not have any penetration of any kind.

There are people who opt for outercourse for safety reasons. They want to avoid the risk of becoming pregnant or contracting a STI. In these cases, you will typically find that for medical reasons, they can't use certain forms of birth control or are undergoing treatment for serious health issues and can't risk pregnancy or infection. Some young adults who are intimidated to ask their parent's or seek out a clinic for protection may opt for this choice as well.

Is Outercourse and Abstinence the Same

This tends to be a bit of a gray area. It really depends on your own personal definitions here. People practice abstinence for different reasons, much like outercourse. Some are not ready to commit to intercourse because they just aren't ready for that level of physical engagement. Some, as mentioned with outercourse, are being treated for medical conditions and have to avoid pregnancy or infection. Abstinence is practiced for religious reasons, too. All that being said, many people who make that choice have emotions and feelings and can choose what limits and boundaries work for them. This is where outercourse and abstinence can overlap. If those who practice it are taught sex equals penetration, you can see how they would have some similarities.

What Can You Do Practicing Outercourse?

Now that we know the definition and boundaries of outercourse vary greatly from one person to the next, we have compiled a list of what activities can fall within these parameters. Keep in mind, what one person deems acceptable may not be okay for someone else.

- **Make out sessions:** Kissing has always been a very powerful tool when becoming intimate with another person. You can feel connected very quickly. Be mindful of the fact you have an entire body to kiss, no need to stick just to the lips.

- **Massage:** Another fabulous way to be connected to your partner. Warm up some massage oil, put on some soft music and light some candles. Do a check-in with your partner to establish boundaries about where they are comfortable being touched.

- **Mutual touching:** As humans we came into this world craving touch and connection. Again, communicate your intentions and check with your partner about boundaries. Inquire about mutual masturbation and if they are okay with this. Achieving orgasm this way may be perfectly acceptable with both partners.

- **Touching yourself:** If you or your partner are not comfortable with mutual masturbation why not try taking turns watching each other. This can also help keep you both connected in a steamy way. Don't forget to bring some lube into the mix to bump the excitement factor up a notch.

- **Dry humping:** I know this is one you may not have thought of since your teen years, but you should absolutely revisit it. Rubbing or grinding up against your partner can bring pleasure in many ways. Yes, this is done with clothes on typically, but that choice is yours. This gives you both a chance to familiarize yourselves with positions you enjoy as well.

- **Toys:** This is a personal choice, but whether you agree to penetration or not, toys are always fun. If you are a hard no on penetration, use these toys to stimulate the nipples, the penis, or any erogenous zone you please. If penetration with toys is okay for you, then make your shopping trip an adventure. Too shy to visit a store? No worries, log on to your favorite store and browse away. They will deliver to you discreetly and you can enjoy it in no time.

- **Oral sex:** Have this discussion with your partner and if you both agree, oral sex can be a wonderful part of outercourse. Using your mouths to explore each other will keep you connected. Don't forget the anus as well!

Are There Any Risks Involved?

When you are in close proximity with another person, there will be risks. Let's break down what we need to be careful of with outercourse.

Pregnancy
Many believe because there is no intercourse involved, there is no chance for pregnancy. This is not true. Yes, we cut the odds way down by eliminating the largest factor,

penis in vagina, but we aren't out of the woods all together. Semen is the key here, and if you are allowing fingering, and semen is on the finger accidentally, this creates a risk. If semen makes contact with the vulva at any time, you run a risk of pregnancy. Things can get steamy, and fluids are everywhere, so yes, be careful. Handwashing after ejaculation will reduce this risk and keep your eyes on that semen.

There have been plenty of cases where couples are practicing outercourse only, but in the heat of the moment, they cannot contain themselves. Hormones are powerful, so please be prepared beforehand and keep condoms on hand.

STIs
Yes, even without having intercourse, you run the risk of transmitting a STI. You just have to remember that anytime you are in contact with bodily fluids and other people's genitals, this is a risk. For example, if you and your partner decide dry humping is acceptable, but you are going to keep your underwear on to be safe. Things get steamy quick, and your underwear is wet, really wet. Those fluids will be in contact with your partner's underwear, which most certainly also have wet spots.

One thing most partners don't think of is sex toys. They can be a breeding ground for STIs if not cleaned properly. A couple is having a great time, sharing those toys back and forth and now their STI is your STI. This is a great reason to keep condoms on hand; sliding one over the toy and peeling it off for your partner is a quick and easy way to keep you both protected.

Both oral and anal sex are significant ways to transmit STIs as well. Infections of the mouth can transfer to the genitals and vice versa. Communicate with your partner before engaging in these activities so you can both continue to be safe and free of infection.

Why Outercourse?

Now, after reading all of this you may be asking yourself why people engage in outercourse when sex is so much better.

It's great to know that there are so many ways to give and receive pleasure. Being physically intimate is a personal decision. How each person decides to engage is up to you. Here are some reasons why you might consider engaging in outercourse.

- You made a critical error and forgot protection. You know you cannot risk infection or pregnancy, so outercourse it is.

- You are respecting your partner's wishes. They are not ready for penetration yet. Their reason could be pain, body image issues, or they just aren't ready yet.

- For those who have chosen to use the birth control method of tracking your cycle, this may be one of your high fertile times. In this case outercourse will help you avoid pregnancy.

- Outercourse is a wonderful way to stay connected if either you or your partner are menstruating and choose not to have sex. When menstruating, you can get pretty frisky from that flood of hormones, and many often have an increased desire to physically connect.

- Some STIs will bring about flare ups of the genitals. It can be embarrassing and painful. It doesn't mean we don't still want to feel physically connected. This is a great time to practice outercourse.

- Why not try outercourse to explore your own body? If you are trying to understand how your own body works, take it slow and introduce your partner when you are ready.

- When starting out a new relationship, we need to learn about each other. Rather than rushing straight to intercourse, this offers us the time to learn what we both like and what works.

- Outercourse is the best solution if either party isn't ready for intercourse. When you are respecting those boundaries but still want that connection, this is your best option. Remember to communicate those boundaries to one another.

- It is quite common for people to have their first sexual experience and it does not go well. They may make a decision then, that they need more time. Engaging in outercourse during this time, is perfect in this situation.

- If you are finding things a little stale in your sexual relationship, why not challenge your partner to "no intercourse" and see what they come up with? They can do anything to you but penetration. Sounds like a fun game to me.

- If the foreplay in your relationship is flat or non-existent, bring outercourse into the mix. Explain the premise to your partner, no penetration allowed. Set a time, a week, a month and maybe see how long you both can go. Imagine the heat and passion when intercourse is reintroduced.

We must keep reminding ourselves that there is more than one way to climb a tree. Whichever way leads you to pleasure, do that. It's healthy to be confident and safe in how you give and receive sexual pleasure.

Self-Pleasure

Jesse Kahn, a licensed psychotherapist and sex therapist based in New York City, explains touch releases oxytocin, reduces stress, and calms our nervous system. The absence of it, he says, can manifest as "depression or anxiety or a feeling of loneliness or stress" (Sethi, 2021).

We have a much greater capacity to bring the comfort of touch to ourselves than we might realize. Celebrating our bodies, and the pleasure they can give us, can be the starting point for an extraordinary relationship with ourselves and the world. Here's how to get started.

If self-exploration is new, treat it like a new relationship with another person: be curious and give it time. "You don't just have to necessarily focus on majorly erogenous zones," Stubbs says. "Touch your earlobe or notice the way your fingers caress your neck." And then, keep going. "You may find that light touch is just enough. Or maybe you want to apply more pressure, a percussive tapping, a tweaking. It's fun to experience different sensations" (Stubbs, 2021).

"Masturbation can be the turning point for a lot of people when it comes to making peace with their bodies," Stubbs writes in her book, *Playing Without a Partner*. "Understanding that you are worthy of sexual pleasure is so powerful. You, in whatever body right now, can and deserve to experience pleasure" (Stubbs, 2021).

I am a true believer in exploring our own bodies. Being comfortable with yourself is the first step to being comfortable with others in any sexual or pleasurable way. Who better to show them what brings you pleasure and climax than you?

For many, penetration alone will not bring about ultimate and heightened pleasure. We all want to have our toes curl as we feel that sexual release, and knowing how to achieve that is crucial. This is why exploration is key.

Foreplay

This is the world of teasing, tempting and intrigue, if you are lucky! Foreplay has gone through many changes over the years, and I believe it just needs better education and focus. We need to put a huge spotlight on the importance of foreplay and the sexual relationships of many would improve overnight.

Why Is It Important?

Foreplay is not just important, it is a link in the pleasure chain we all need. I like to compare any human body to a car attempting to start on a freezing cold day. I know for me; I jump in, start it up, and turn the heat on. I impatiently wait for that warm air to defrost the windows and get me hot. I have been known to talk nicely to my car to warm up my buns. Cars do not drive optimally when cold and stiff. They need time to warm up; the engine is cold, so it can't be expected to operate at its peak the minute I demand it to. Do you see where I'm headed with this? Genitals are much like a car engine. You cannot expect to hop on your partner, booty-call or spouse and get right to work. The vagina needs lubrication, and for that to happen, foreplay is necessary. Many of us are psychological beings, so to get those juices flowing, you need time and teasing. Some of us are visual beings, so you too need to see temptation and desire for arousal to stimulate your fun parts. So, what exactly constitutes foreplay, you ask? Great question, because trust me, one kiss on the neck and a tweak of the nipple isn't going to cut it. Even my car demands more than a minute for that heat to come on.

Great Foreplay Ideas

Let's get started discussing some great ways to heat up everyone's engines. Feel free to adapt any of these ideas to your particular situation.

Reminisce About the Past

Hear me out on this one. You are sitting around eating a delicious meal and your topic of dinner conversation turns to "days gone by." Bring up all those hot spots you've had sex, or crazy positions you tried. There is something about connecting yourselves to the past that fuels the body to want to relive them again. Be specific in your conversation, recall what you were wearing and how hot the sex was.

Stay Out of the Bedroom

Why not begin the teasing well before the final curtain? Is your partner cooking dinner? Why not move in behind them in the kitchen and whisper your intentions for later on? Be specific about what you want to do to them and walk away. Is your partner upstairs working in their office? Send a risky photo with instructions about what you plan to do later. Again, the details matter, so be specific.

Set the Scene

A common complaint is that there is never any thought put into foreplay, so it gets stale. Plan ahead and get that bucket of ice, or that candle for wax play. Why not create your go to foreplay kit and keep it in a place close to your bed, or on a closet shelf if you have wee ones. Create this kit when you are feeling super horny; that way it is truly inspired with sex in mind. That way, if it has been a crazy week, you aren't standing in the room with zero capacity to be creative. Just grab your foreplay kit and enjoy. Add your blindfold, handcuffs, lube, paddle, whatever you both enjoy should be in this kit.

Who Wants to Dance?

Now this may be reserved for those special occasions, birthdays, Wednesdays, whichever. Putting together a sexy dance for your partner will have them wanting to rip those clothes off you. I mention clothes, because our brains love mystery. Don't come *Full Monty* right out the gate. Peel those layers slowly and let your anticipation build.

Lay Down Rules

Whenever there is an extra layer of intrigue, it builds sexual tension. Try whispering to your partner, while you are licking the nipples, or barely touching the genitals, that they have to be super quiet, or they can't kiss you. Better yet, tell them they can't touch any part of your body, get naked and hover over them while getting them close to climax; it will send them so close to the edge, they will be begging you.

Massages? Yes Please!

We are all exhausted living our best life, so who on earth is going to turn down a massage? The best sensual massages are all about setting the mood. We don't want three quick neck rubs and then be expected to hop on top. Light those candles, make sure the room isn't too hot or too cold, and a little mood music would be wonderful. To heighten this game, ask if they wouldn't mind being blindfolded. As you have their naked body covered in warm massage oil—yes, you should warm it up—and they can't see you, brush your hard penis against their leg, or let your breasts graze their back. Sensual massages are amazing foreplay for both partners. Just do your best to focus on a really great massage, and before too long, you will both be coated in warm massage oil and climaxing with passion.

Want to Watch a Movie?
When was the last time you both watched a really hot movie together? If you leave your inhibitions at the door, this can be one topic of foreplay that gets you hot and ready quickly. Watching people perform oral sex on each other can make you feel twinges in your own genitals. You may even find some new positions to try.

Okay, keeping in mind this is just a beginner's list, it will be something to get you started. When and if you are comfortable, don't forget to bring in all those amazing toys you are going to read about in this chapter. The sexual world is your oyster and what a world it is.

Exploring Sexual Pleasure Together

While you set the stage for your exploration, you should be keeping all of your senses in mind. The ability to heighten all of them will be a game changer. I have listed a few ideas below to get you started.

- **A blindfold**. Taking away your sight heightens your sense of touch. Feel the goosebumps form on your skin as your partner (or you) slides different textures across your body. It also heightens your sense of hearing. Tune in to their change in breathing as they get excited. Pay close attention to your own as well. Listen closely to your surroundings.

- **Music**. Some are easily distracted by the sounds of the world. Put on soothing, calm music and watch the difference. You will feel your muscles relax and your body will be more conducive to pleasure. You can also use slow music or songs that have a pounding and rhythmic tempo you can kiss, rub, lick, finger, nibble, suck and stroke to.

- **Erotic massage**. Physical human touch is powerful. Allowing your partner to coat your naked body in warm massage oil and then massage your breasts, inner thighs, or buttocks will have you experiencing pleasure you didn't know existed. For heightened pleasure, keep on that blindfold and let that music play.

- **Light spanking**. People become intrigued with spanking for a few reasons. First, it awakens the feelings of sexual touch. It intensifies the feeling of touch and the responsiveness to pleasure. You can use just the palm of your hand, or you can branch out into paddles, riding crops, or floggers. Spanking can be used during foreplay or intercourse, and there is no need to overthink it. Have a discussion with your partner and establish a safe word. Once you are both comfortable, experiment in a safe environment and enjoy.

- **Take it outside**. Don't get arrested, but having sex in public is a fantasy for many people. Wendasha Jenkins Hall, Ph.D., a sex educator, and researcher says, "People like it because there's the possibility and the thrill of getting caught."(Jenkins, 2020) You have to be careful, though, because each city and jurisdiction has its own laws about public indecency, Jenkins Hall advises. Pro tip: Stay in your car or go into a secluded place at dusk to keep yourself away from potential viewers, and then... get your freak on!

- **Temperature play**. This is a fantastic way to spice up your pleasure level that not many think of. Incorporate temperature play into the bedroom. Try classic techniques like grabbing an ice cube and gently running it up and down each other's bodies. Then blow hot air onto each other's inner thighs, with deep inhale and exhale breaths. In short, the various temps bring a new physical sensation to sex that you might not have experienced before.

- **Fingering**. It is time to let your fingers do the walking. Digital stimulation can be an amazing tool for pleasure. Whether you are pleasuring yourself or someone else, this is all about reading the room and taking your time. If you are with a partner, it is going to be very important to pay attention to their reactions. If you are exploring with your fingers and you get a reaction, take note. There is also zero need to head straight for the honey pot. Let's take our time here and tease. Circle those testicles, trace the shaft, lightly trail your finger down the labia, and circle those nipples. Oftentimes, we feel the need to get to the end goal quickly; I am here to tell you the journey is just as fun as the happy ending. Digital stimulation is wonderful for the clitoris, the penis, nipples and the anus. Take your time and find out where your sweet spots are.

- **Palming**. For some of you who may not be aware of this technique, I am going to try to break it down for you. This one is all about the vagina. The intent is to stimulate not only the clitoris, but all the goodness around it as well. This technique gets its name because the actual palm of the hand is used on the clitoris. Two fingers will be inserted into the vagina. This will be the ring and middle fingers. These fingers will put pressure against the upper vaginal wall while sliding in and out, gaining a good rhythm. The rest of the fingers on the hand will be fully extended. You can hold on to them, or they can rest on the thigh. This can be done to yourself or have another person give it a try. Be patient, go slow at first, but when you are successful, this will be a unique orgasm you will be sure to enjoy.

- **Rimming**. The anus is one of the body parts that holds one of the highest amounts of nerve endings. Rimming, also known as analingus is one of the more common forms of non-penetrative forms of anal pleasure play. In its basic form, rimming is oral sex for the anus. You are using your mouth, lips, or tongue to apply pleasurable sensations to your partner's anus. If you are just getting started with exploring the anus, this is a great place to start. It is not invasive and tends to be less intimidating for that reason.

- **Naked dry humping**. This is just the act of humping, minus the act of penetration of any kind. Dry humping may not be high on the list of hot sex acts and it can be far from elegant, but trust me, it can be extremely sexually gratifying. Is there the possibility of some awkward bending and twisting? Yes. Could you be accidentally tossed from the bed? Maybe? But hey, it is what you make it. You have the option of keeping your clothes on (for those feeling a bit shy), dressing a bit naughty, or naked as a jaybird. The positioning is all up to you as well. Sit, lay down, squat, whichever is going to get the job done. There is no wrong way to do this. The name of the game is rubbing your genitals against yourself, or a partner, in absolutely any position that feels fantastic. Bonus, if you are flying solo, you can completely do this by yourself. Grab a cozy pillow, or an upholstered piece of furniture and go to town.

- **Sexy showers**. Have you ever been surprised by your partner jumping in that hot shower with you? Shower sex can be sexy and invigorating. The water trickling down their skin, the moist steam fogging up the glass, the clean, delicious smells floating in the air, and that wet, naked skin. Now, can we be real for a moment? Shower sex has its challenges. The temperature has to be just right. And, nobody wants to be sitting in the emergency room for hours because the slippery conditions have us elevating a broken ankle. The nurses will love the story, though. The name of the game with shower sex is safety first. Rinse the floor of all soaps and suds to prevent those falls. Lastly, just be sure those positions are secure before getting too hot and heavy.

- **Cunnilingus**. Conversations surrounding oral sex and the vagina usually involve those who will spend years researching and mastering the craft, and those who do not. The one thing we know for certain is that no two people have the same clitoral response. So, no two techniques will work the same. What is the best way to please a vagina, then? Communication. Yes, that is right; talk first. Ask your partner what they enjoy, what works and what does not. If nobody has ever asked them, take this opportunity to go slow, try some things and get a thumbs up or down. The other big mistake that is often made here is there is no lead up. X marks the spot; there is the bullseye and nothing else matters. Nobody wants to start that car when it is minus thirty out; no one really enjoys aggressive clitoral stimulation the minute they expose it. Tease, taunt, explore, and both of your experiences will be better for it. There are some great things you can incorporate to up your game. Ask them to pull your hair if they enjoy what you are trying. Some people can be self-conscious about their vagina health, so toss out a few remarks about how great they taste for reassurance. Don't be afraid to use those hands as well, try nipple stimulation, or go for that g-spot.

- **Vaginal hood oral sex**. To begin, let's be sure everyone knows the location of the vaginal "hood." Also called the clitoral hood, it is, quite literally, a flap at the top of the vagina that covers the external clitoris. You can think of it much as foreskin protects a penis if it's not circumcised. Now, onto why this little gem could be your best friend. For many, if you begin oral sex by lifting the hood and making direct contact with the clitoris, it will be way too much stimulation. Instead, leave the hood right where it is and stimulate the clitoris over the said hood. Right? Genius at work here. Once you're in the groove a bit more here you can lift the hood and maybe blow gently on the clitoris and gauge their reaction. If they're giving you all the green light signals, you may proceed.

- **Fellatio**. The one thing I have observed over the years is people either love giving blow jobs or hate it. The first step to changing this mindset is to stop thinking of it as a job. When done correctly, it should be explosive and pleasurable for you both. This is a production and should be treated as such. There is no need to rip back the covers and put that penis in your mouth. Tease it until they can't handle it any longer. You want them to feel your breath on their inner thighs, stomach, and testicles. Run your fingernails lightly across their skin. Maintain eye contact with them as you lightly run your lips across the shaft of the penis. Watch for those cues, and notice their breathing change. Suggest blindfolding to heighten the senses even more. Bust out that lube, the market offers lots of flavored options, so pick the one you will enjoy licking off the head of their erection. Start it slow. Then progress and quicken your speed, especially as they begins to react. The slower and more intensely you go, the more they'll react. You want that tease game to be on point. It is a misconception that you have to do this at the speed of light. You also do not need to be deep-throating the penis the entire time. There are plenty of erogenous zones up and down the shaft and on the head; find them and tease those too. Grip the base of their penis and use your hands in a rhythmic motion to help. Be sure you are showing them how much you are enjoying this, too. Many are visual and watching you becoming turned on will add to the arousal. Lastly, be sure to discuss any boundaries ahead of time. Some people are not comfortable with deep-throating or having someone finish in their mouth. These are all healthy boundaries, just be clear to discuss them before you are in the heat of it all.

The Sex Position Bucket List

We all have our favorite, don't we? We will make reservations a month ahead of time to get a table at our favorite restaurant. We leave early for work every day to grab our favorite coffee. We never miss an episode of our favorite television show. So, when it comes to sex positions, we can have a favorite, but it is great to have an arsenal to pull from. Nobody enjoys being boring and mundane between the sheets.

Be mindful of the fact that it isn't just your body having sex, your brain is too. It is a huge part of this equation, and it needs stimulating as much as your genitals. If you stick to those same two moves, it is likely to shut down and then you are fighting to stay awake.

When couples start to notice their sex life take a turn for the worst, they need to communicate why. They may be shocked to find out pain is an issue. There are some who experience painful intercourse for many reasons. Chronic pain sufferers hurt everywhere, and others have gynecological issues and suffer in silence. Finding suitable sex positions can bring joy back into your sex life and not have to miss out on having orgasms and pleasure. That being said, there are more sex positions available than stars in the sky. Okay maybe not quite, but there are a lot. Below, you will find the top five on many lists.

- **The 69**. Let's visit this position first. Many can be extremely self-conscious of this position, as it leaves you pretty vulnerable. This is not the go to position straight out of the gym. Have a nice shower together first if that eases your anxiety. Your partner should be on their back, then you will climb on top with your face in their genitals, basically. Each partner should be lined up, face to genitals. You can also do the 69 laying on your side, it's a little less physically intimidating. Yes, this is for oral sex and a good foreplay position, but don't shy away from bringing in a toy.

- **The valedictorian**. You can start with one partner on their back and the other hovering over their body in between their legs. You take your receiving partner's legs and spread them wide, like the letter V and place their calves on your shoulders. Depending on flexibility, you can make their legs bend or straight. If you're working with a vagina, you can grab your partners bum to add more friction for your clitoral stimulation.

- **The corkscrew**. You will want to pull yourself as close to the bed as possible, resting on your forearm and hip (so, laying on your side). In this position, your thighs should be together. Your partner will be standing on the floor behind you to enter or kneeling on the bed. If you keep those thighs nice and tight, it creates a wonderful feeling for your partner and you. Get proactive in your pleasure and guide your partner's hand to your arousal points for more stimulation.

- **Bamboo splitter.** One partner is laying on their back and with one leg down and one leg spread with a bent knee. Your partner is in between your legs and can enter inside you. They are propped up by having one arm by your right shoulder and one arm holding your bent leg over their right shoulder. Switch up legs and arms of course and even try blind folded.

- **The face-off**. No, we aren't about to play naked hockey. Bring a chair into the bedroom and drape it with a towel or sheet for easy clean-up. Have your partner sit on the edge. You should now straddle them, facing them on their lap. It will be easier for you to have your knees up or squat depending on your comfort level. You now have full control over penetration level and speed.

- **The spider legs.** One partner is sitting half way up on their elbows and the other is laying on their back with legs open and feet are in between your partner. With your strap on or penis, meet up in the middle for rubbing, rimming, or stroking. Set a nice rhythm by rocking back and forth. As always, reach over and touch your partner or yourself as you make eye contact.

- **The doggy style**. You should be on all fours, and I always recommend this on a bed or cushy flooring, as the bare floor will make your knees sore in a hurry. Nobody wants to rush this. Once you are in position, have your partner get behind you. This is a fantastic position for locating that G-spot and deep anal and vaginal penetration. Don't forget that you can ask your partner to find your sensitive parts and add some layers to this party.

- **The flatiron**. You will want to lay flat on your stomach on the bed, again comfort will be key. Your hips should be slightly raised (use those core muscles) and legs should be straight. Now, your partner needs to be on top entering from behind. This is an amazing position if your partner has a smaller penis, or you are using a strap-on. It creates a tight fit, so everything stays put.

- **The side by side.** Think spooning each other but being front to front. You can make eye contact with your partner and kiss. One partner lifts a leg to allow access for the strap on or penis to enter and use your knees, feet and the ability to hold each other to build some pleasurable, friction filled thrusts.

Great Sex Positions for a Great Orgasm

Public Service Announcement! For those partners who want to give their women and vagina-owners an orgasm. Patience is the name of the game. Working for the first orgasm may take the longest amount of time. However, subsequent climaxes tend to come a lot quicker. Stay in the game.

We know that if achieving an orgasm is your goal as a vagina-haver, clitoral friction is your friend. Sex positions that naturally cause bodies to rub together or the vagina to make contact with a nice gentle surface can help you get your pleasure fix. So, if you're not in this type of sex position, just do it yourself. Use your fingers and self-pleasure while you're being penetrated. You certainly know how to, right? It's hot and gets the job done. Depending on the position, your partner can use their fingers, or palm while stroking away, and don't forget about bringing a vibrator to the party. This is also a win-win because your partner will get to see you climax and be turned on by your eroticism.

Here are five tried and true orgasmic-filled positions. Try them all out. See which ones work best for you and yours.

- **The Lotus.** This is probably one of the most intimate and romantic sex positions. It requires both partners to sit straddled onto each other. The penetrating partner on the bottom and receiving partner on the top. The penetrating partner is either crossed legged or sitting with legs straight out and partner on top while sitting on top of your partner's parts. Face to face. Arms around each other. Start to work together to develop a pleasurable rhythm and make any adjustments to reach for an internal climax.

- **The Spoons.** A classic position that is always lovely first thing in the morning. It's great because you're not facing your partner and don't have to worry as much about morning breath. It's also a great position for those who might feel more conscious about their body size. Laying back to front with your receiving partner, you enter your partner from behind, while on your side. You can rub on their wet and hardened parts at the same time or take turns, squeeze on breasts, kiss and caress until your time has come.

- **The Chilled-out Rider.** This is the sexy and empowering position that many women and vulva-owners enjoy. As the receiver, straddle your partner while they lay down with legs stretched straight out. Focus your attention on grinding on the penis or dildo for greater pleasure. Riding up and down is fine if it's your preference, but for many, it can be too intense, painful and not create any real clitoral stimulation. Grinding, on the other hand, can be further heightened by leaning back a bit while in motion. Leaning back can also engage your g-spot stimulation. Your partner can take it even further by gently stroking their fingers on your clitoris to bring you over the edge.

- **The Pin-down.** As a receiving partner, you're laying down on the bed, or couch. Your penetrating partner will lay on top of you from behind and insert. This is a great position for a vagina-haver as you can naturally receive great pleasure both from your partner's strokes, as well as the friction from the surface you're lying on. You can use your fingers or a comfortable vibrator. Also consider using a small pillow or blanket to help elevate the pelvis.

- **The Missionary 2.0.** This position is commonly known as the Coital Alignment Technique or CAT. It has been known to have pretty reliable results with many women who've reached climax while in this position. It's a great clitoral stimulator. Here's the set up. As the receiving partner, lay down on your back, preferably with a small pillow or blanket below your bottom. Your penetrating partner then mounts you similarly to the missionary position, but the difference is that your partner needs to shift their body up for several inches. Your penetrating partner should aim to have their chest near your shoulders. Keep each other close to encourage good friction from the penis shaft to the vulva and clitoris. Trust me on this one, it will be a winner for all involved.

Hopefully this list will be just a start for you as you seek to expand your sexual creativity and pleasure. There's so much more to learn, explore and discover. Get to it!

Lesbians Are Having Great Sex

Lesbians are achieving much higher levels of sexual pleasure and satisfaction in surveys than women who have sex with men.

A Public Health England survey of more than 7,000 women found that half of respondents aged between 25 and 34 reported their sex life has been disappointing. The percentage dropped to 29% among 55 to 64-year-olds, proving sex for women improves with age (Public Health England, 2018).

A 2014 study by the Journal of Sexual Medicine found that lesbians orgasmed 75% of the time during sex, compared with 61% for heterosexual women (Garcia et al., 2014).

The burning question on everyone's mind is... how is heterosexual sex missing the orgasm mark and lesbian sex right on target? Lesbians know their body, they know where the clitoris is and how to manipulate it to achieve orgasm. No time is wasted showing their partner what to do. No frustration or ego petting required, because clearly, their partner has the same parts. Emotionally, they tend to be on the same page, knowing how women require foreplay and emotional attachment, these partners know how to feed into every part of sex.

When a woman has sex with another woman, it's a completely mind-altering experience. It is a tender mix of romance, love, emotion and intensity. At the end of the day, women have the best and hottest sex with other women because they understand each other physically and emotionally. They communicate their needs, zone in on the hot areas like the clitoris, focus less on penetration, and aim to please. Take notes folks.

GGG

GGG stands for 'good, giving, and game'. Sex advice columnist Dan Savage developed the concept otherwise known as GGG. It describes a person who has no problem expressing their sexuality and is willing to try new things sexually. So they are 'good' at communicating their sexual desires and needs, have no qualms 'giving' or satisfying their partner's needs and is willing or 'game' to anything new. Based on the GGG approach, each of us should all be striving to become 'good, giving and game' in order to have the most satisfying sexual experiences. GGG has overtime become a sex positive term and even incorporated on many dating apps as a way for individuals to express this as a part of their own identity.

According to Katherine Peach, wellness blogger,

> The GGG approach is centered around both partners finding sexual satisfaction, regardless if a partner shares the same turn on or kink. Savage is quick to emphasize sexual acts shouldn't turn someone off or make them feel violated. Instead, the goal of GGG is reciprocation by working toward more enjoyment and avoiding resentment for not having your needs met. GGG can be especially helpful for long-term, committed relationships where one person is expected to fulfill as much of their partner's needs as possible (Peach, 2021).

I think we can all appreciate being with someone who is dedicated to giving you pleasure. Someone who is at least willing to try, within reason, to make you feel good. In fact, scientific research outlined in the *Social Psychological and Personality Science* journal found that in a sample of individuals in a relationship 'people [with] sexual communal strength (i.e., those motivated to meet a romantic partner's sexual needs) have partners who are more satisfied with and committed to their relationships (Muise and Impett, 2014). Now that sounds like finding a pot of gold at the end of a rainbow! Count me in!

Researchers at the University of Toronto performed a study in 2012 to see if the GGG mentality showed positive or negative impacts on sexual satisfaction for couples. Amy Muise, Ph.D., one of the researchers explains that,

> In a sample of long-term couples (together for 11 years on average), we found people who were higher in sexual communal strength reported higher levels of daily sexual desire and were more likely to maintain their desire over time. People who began the study with high sexual communal strength-maintained desire over a 4-month period, whereas those who started off low in sexual communal strength saw a decline in their sexual desire (Muise, 2012).

Now, when it comes to research studies, it's important to remember there can be other factors that may play into why people decide to remain committed and maintain sexual desire. But hopefully you can appreciate that there's something to be said about being willing to attend to your partner's sexual needs and desires. It's important not to overthink the approach here. The main driver is being open and having a willingness to please your partner and be pleased. However you and your partner decide this should look like is all up to you. It's supposed to be a win-win situation.

Being good at GGG is also about meeting your own needs. If we unpack what it means to have 'sexual communal strength', it's really talking about being motivated to give pleasure, not by force or through guilt but feeling good about yourself for satisfying your partner. If my partner wants me to dress up in a pleather cat suit while being flogged on my knees, I personally find it empowering. My partner desires me and sees me as sexy and wants me. It's not coming from a place of wanting to demean me, but to play a sexy role that leads to further sexual intimacy. I feel emboldened and powerful turning my partner on and driving them wild with arousal. This in turn makes me want them even more.

I think being good at communicating what you want sexually should be classified as a life skill. It's not as simple as it seems. We all know the common saying, it's better to give than receive', right? For some, thinking of articulating where and how you feel pleasure is embarrassing and can bring about feelings of shame and shyness. But it doesn't have to be. With practice, you can shed your bashfulness and feel more comfortable. I personally, didn't spend enough time thinking about how I wanted to be pleased and what brought me great pleasure so it was difficult. I had to spend time pleasuring myself, trying different sex toys on my own before starting to put my mind on voicing what pleases me. Having a partner who is encouraging and excited to please you is definitely helpful. Having a pleasure cheerleader is a great way to help you detail what you need sexually.

To help get you started with becoming good at communicating your needs, start with an action that would be easier for you to describe. For instance, ask your partner for a foot massage. During your massage, keep eye contact and describe to your partner how it feels. Provide directions on speed, intensity, direction and location of where they move their hands. Tell them when it feels good. Tell them when it feels rea-lly good. Next time try another part of your body and see how you feel giving direction of how you want to be pleasured, allow your partner to respond and go from there.

Say thank you. Yes, you can't go wrong with expressing gratitude to your partner for prioritizing your pleasure. Katherine Peach also explains that 'expressing gratitude to your partner has shown to increase how much communal strength participants saw in their relationship, which makes for stronger relationships overall'. It seems like a no brainer to say thank you but when in a relationship, sometimes we can take kindness for granted but gratitude will always be worth it. So, keep an open mind when you're talking with your partner. In the next few chapters, I'll be discussing a myriad of sexual toys, activities and tools to keep your sexual connections on fire.

CHAPTER 5: Tools and Toys to Elevate Pleasure

"People see my kindle and all they see is an e-reader. I see a sex toy" - **Alexis Angel**

The pleasure enhancement market has been on the rise, but what most are not aware of is that it is exploding… pun intended. The sexual wellness market is on target to reach US$45.05 billion by 2026 (Markets, 2021). It is important to note that this boom is on a global scale. So, who can tell us why we are spending so much money on sex?

There is no mistaking that there is a new sexual culture in town. Its name is to hell with stigma and it is here to stay. Across all cultures, we are fed up with sex shaming. More of us want to live a life of love, sex, and pleasure, without being judged. This is now allowing us to explore, change attitudes, and finally link sexual wellness into our everyday life.

There are four more major contributing factors to this massive growth in the pleasure enhancement market (Markets, 2021), they include:

- growth of the digital marketplace
- an uptick in the usage of dating apps in Asian/Pacific countries

- increase due to sexual wellness fairs, trade shows, and expos, and

- huge growth in government initiatives for free condom distribution worldwide.

Where is the Money Going?

Now we can get an even closer picture of the money by breaking down these statistics even further. Let's get a more concise overview of the billions people are sinking into the pleasure industry.

- Condoms can account for just over 99% of the entire global market.

- International vendors are finally getting their day in the sun. Due to massive development within the infrastructure and the boom in research and development, they are now able to expand their presence in the market.

- North America is solid in the already developed sexual wellness empire. That being said, it is forecasted to reach $10.50 billion by 2026.

- Sex toys are the leader. In 2020, they led the market. They held a strong market share of 57.71%. The interesting twist is that sex toys are now seeing a massive demand from places like China and Japan.

So, welcome to the world of pleasure. In this chapter we are going to cover the entire world of external tools and toys you can bring into your world to enhance your pleasure game. These are intended to help you reach all your happy endings. It makes no difference if you are alone or with a partner or two. Use this time to experiment and explore your body and that of a partner.

Most Popular Sexual Pleasure Tools

Sex toys now are not what they used to be like. You could order them from sex shops or even in department stores but they would never clearly say what the purpose was for. 'Personal massager' was a common name for vibrators back then and they were often the first pleasure tool for most several generations ago. They resembled a fat, white, candlestick one might find on their grandmother's dining room table. They were hard plastic, and it held four D batteries. If you powered them on for any longer than three minutes, they would burn your hand. And, they sounded as if you were mowing your neighbor's lawn under the blankets! Yes, we have definitely come a long way.

Sex-tech, has been making a real name for itself in the pleasure market over the last ten years. We have actual sex toy experts. They design our toys from a pleasure and medical point of view. Every single one of us walking this earth is finally getting the sex toys we have been yearning for and desire. They are softer, silkier, and quieter. No more rummaging through drawers to find a good battery to finish that orgasm. These beauties are USB chargeable, yep just like your phone.

New and exciting toys to explore for everyone. But before we get too deep into all the new and exciting toys we have to explore, let's take a quick second to explore erogenous zones. Let's face it, we need to know where to point for pleasure.

The vulva. This is the entire exterior of the vagina encompassing the clitoris, the urethra, and both labia—minora and majora.

The clitoris. The clitoris is much larger than most realize. It is not just what you visually see on the exterior. Internally, it runs down both sides of the vagina, which leads you to the G-spot.

The nipple. Most of us have two of them, so we can double our pleasure. Titillating the nipples can create strong sexual arousal with our human parts. They can also bring about much pleasure with sex toys like nipple clamps, pumps, suckers and cups.

The penis. The shaft of the penis is actually called the phallus and it has two fun zones. The top of the shaft, or the phallus, is called the glans. This is what most refer to as the head of the penis. On the underside of the head of the penis is a thin piece of connective tissue, this is called the frenulum. This is extremely sensitive when stimulated.

The anus. Yes, the butthole. Not to be confused with the rectum, which is the interior portion, and that is what attaches to the anus. Don't be afraid to do your research on both of these areas. Knowledge is pleasure, and once you have the information, you will feel both safe and educated to explore. These areas are very sensitive and can be pleasurable with internal and external stimulation.

The prostate. If you have a penis, there's an additional erogenous zone here: the prostate or P-spot. A walnut-sized gland between the internal structures of the penis and the rectum. It can be reached by toys that curve toward the front of your body.

The toes. If feet and toes are your thing sexually there is also good and pleasurable sensations to be had down there. Try out toe suckers or even fake feet to get you going.

There you have it, the why, where and how. Now, let's move on to the what!

External Pleasure Tools

Now that we have looked at ways we can enhance pleasure with just our bodies and some creativity, let's take a walk into the world of what is available on the pleasure market.

Whichever creative way you decide to bring these items into your life, always remember, your end goal here is joy, pleasure and orgasms, lots and lots of orgasms. Spend as much time as you want or wish experimenting with these alone. When or if you wish, invite someone in to explore with you. Establish your rules and safe words if necessary. Keep in mind that having trust between people will heighten that pleasure level.

Sex Toy Staples

- **Vibrators**. The vibrator industry is hawt! There are so many varieties of vibrators on the market right now to soothe and relieve your sexual tension. As sexual wellness starts to become recognized as a part of our greater holistic health, more mainstream retail outlets are starting to sell them. To be honest, my last trip to the adult store had me holding a sex toy in awe of how much it resembled my electric toothbrush! You can find small ones, large ones, double-sided, flower-shaped, rabbit-shaped, curvy, or in wand form. Vibrators are great to be used solo or with a partner. Just be mindful that some can be very intense on the sensitive spots on our bodies. Once you find the rhythm and speed that brings you into ecstasy, be sure to add many to your daily life routine.

Dildos

- **Glass Dildos**. Glass vs silicone, the great debate. Those who have traveled over to the glass side swear they will never go back, so why? Glass is easy to clean, no fancy cleaners necessary, just good old-fashioned soap and water. If temperature play is your thing, glass is perfect. These are constructed to tolerate super cold or super-hot conditions. Just test on your wrist before using on any sensitive body part. Typically, designed with bulbous ends, they are perfect for any type of anal play. Did we mention how beautifully stunning they are? Already smooth to the touch, add a dollop of lube and it is party time. Glass is also hypoallergenic for those who struggle with sensitivities to many of the silicones used in other vibrators. If you are like me and immediately thought, "What happens if this thing shatters?" No worries, they are constructed with Pyrex glass, making them shatterproof. The only thing glass dildos are not recommended for is when using a strap-on. One misguided plunge with a rock hard dildo could result in a big ouch.

- **Double Dildos**. Double dildos might initially seem a bit daunting to some. According to a recent Instagram poll taken by Well+Good, out of 1,400 participants, 76% indicated that they are either very interested in, or have already participated in, double penetration (Kassel, 2022). Double-ended dildos might be worth a try if you want to have some mutual penetration and satisfaction. Compare how you like the toy with your partner. If you are new to this, do your research and take it slow. Also try different positions out for size to see which ones work best with this kind of toy. You can go with your standard, 12-inch, two-headed dildo, and work your way up to those that vibrate and work all the angles.

- **Strap-ons**. A strap-on is a harness and a dildo of your choice. It usually is a combination pack used for penetration. These are typically worn in front of your genitals, simulating a penis. Your options are endless with this wonderful invention. Why not give pegging or good old strap-on sex a try. Keep in mind, strap-on fun is meant to be pleasurable for both the wearer and the recipient. If the one wearing the strap-on has a vagina, they will feel the base of the dildo pressing against the clitoris or pubic mount each time they push.

- **Teledildonics.** Teledildonics is the term used to describe sex toys that can be controlled by another device such as an app or external remote. If you're using these sex toys with a partner, they can control speed and intensity of the vibration on your pleasure parts with a simple press of a button or swipe. So you'll want to mix things up between human pleasure tools like your tongue, hands and genitals and also throw in teledildonics to heighten your partner's pleasure through a device. You can't go wrong with more options to provide pleasure.

   What's even more incredible with teledildonics is the extensive range it possesses for you to control this toy. And, some devices are so smart that you can create and save your own pleasure routine for yourself or your partner. If they like to start off slow and deep and pick up the pace as they start to reach climax keep that winning routine saved for next time. Some teledildonics come with an alarm clock and some even come with music. Others can track the best orgasmic experiences you've had and allow you to send messages back and forth with your partner. So if you and your boo are in a long-distance relationship or just live apart, you can be pleased by your partner while on the phone or on a video chat. Seeing your partner become aroused and sexually undone by your control is hot!

- Let me set the scene for you, you're apart from your boo and send an online meeting request for a one on one meeting at 10pm. The meeting equipment requirements are a bed, blindfold, and your 'special device'. You both sign in to the video meeting while in bed. You ask your mate to position their special device on their pleasure spot and then put on their blindfold. You open your teledildonic device's app and choose how you want to pleasure your partner. Watch them squirm as they start reacting to you. Hear them start moaning as the intensity elevates their pleasure until they are overflowing with ecstasy. Talk dirty to them and encourage them to get their pleasure fix and of course, join in too.

Anal Toys

The anus, the body part we all have and some get a bit squeamish around. It is filled with pleasurable nerve endings, and when done right, you will be glad you explored. Anal toys are designed for us all, from beginner to seasoned pro, you can find something to level up your sex game. I am going to break down the top three leading anal toys and why they have made the list.

b-Vibe Rimming Plug 2.
- Nicknamed the world's first rimming plug, this anal toy is a favorite of Rachel Sommer, Ph.D., a clinical sexologist and founder of *My Sex Toy Guide*.

"It contains rotating beads at the neck, successfully mimicking the feeling of getting your butt licked. This USB rechargeable plug boasts seven modes for the rotating beads and six rotation and vibration intensities, allowing you to regulate the sensations," she says. "Another outstanding feature is the splashproof factor, which allows you to enjoy the plug in the shower"(Sommer, PhD, 2022).

nJoy Pure Wand.
- Introducing a stainless-steel wand. Featuring not one, but two bulbous ends to it and they both offer different sensations. They even managed to weight each end uniquely, which applies pressure to the exact spots needed. Meant to inspire mind-blowing orgasms. Don't forget to get creative and use this toy for temperature play. Simply put it in the fridge or run it under a stream of hot or cold water to open up your world of new sensations.

Booty Sparks 7X Light Up Rechargeable Anal Plug.
- Sexologist Goody Howard, recommends this playful addition to the bedroom. "My favorite anal toy of 2021 is hands down the Booty Sparks rechargeable, waterproof, body-safe, remote control, LED light-up butt plug!" she says. "It

comes in three sizes, so there is a perfect fit no matter how new (or true) you are to anal play. I suggest adding this toy to receiving (or performing) cunnilingus or fellatio and during insertive vaginal sex for an added sense of pressure... and pleasure"(Boom, 2021).

Keep in mind, these are just the top three anal toys, but the list available is vast. It can be overwhelming, so taking it slow and doing research is always recommended. There is a world of butt plugs, anal beads, and prostate massagers just waiting to be discovered.

- **Male masturbation sleeve.** Whether it be an oral sex simulator or a vibration sleeve, these masturbation toys for the penis can be very pleasurable. Most of these toys can be used solo or with a partner to replicate a good stroke, suck, lick and pump. These well designed toys can help you climax without having to do the manual work. You can find them as silicone based, studded, ribbed or smooth all for your intensified pleasure.

- **Lubrication**. People, we need to talk. I do not feel like lube gets enough of a spotlight when it comes to pleasure. So, if you haven't tried it yet, I am here, begging you to spoil yourself right this minute and grab a bottle. Lube is universal to every single body. You can use it with someone or alone. It just makes every single bit of sexual intimacy better. Fun fact, it is also helpful in preventing some sexually transmitted infections and diseases. If you are having intercourse without enough lubrication, you can actually cause small tears or irritation, causing infection to occur more often. There are five types of lubes on the market. Water, silicone, petroleum, oil, and a hybrid-based lubricant. You always want to be mindful of using those water based lubes if you are using condoms. Nobody wants that surprise of a lubricant that eats right through a condom. Yes, this can happen. Now, if you haven't yet tried a lube in the shower... you are missing out. If your brain is trying to map this out, let me help. You want to go with a silicone-based lube in this situation, so the water doesn't just wash it away, but trust me on this, the steamy shower, the slippery genitals, it is hot. It is highly recommended to use lube for any and all anal play, penetration or not. A silicone lubricant works well here, as it is stickier and doesn't dissipate as quickly. A generous amount will help whether you are rimming, fingering, or massaging. If you truly want to up your game, grab some Cannabidiol or CBD lube. This will act as a vasodilator, bringing more blood to the area, decreasing discomfort, and upping your pleasure level.

Other Fun Sex Toys

- **C-rings**. Considered to be the "hot sauce" of men's sex toys, for those who have tried them, they will tell you, all sex is better with a cock ring or c-ring. Typically, a stretchy silicone ring made to go fit around the base of the penis. The intention here is to allow blood to flow into the penis as you become aroused, but restrict blood flow from leaving too easily. The end result is a rock hard penis that is more sensitive, and an erection that can last. Research has shown us that these rings can produce much stronger orgasms. This is achieved by delaying ejaculation causing the intense climax (Nast, 2022).

If you are looking for a c-ring that will please both you and your partner, there are plenty that come with fun textures they can rub up against or built in vibrators. This is a pleasure toy that is great for beginners who want to explore sex toys, but are a bit intimidated by some of the others.

- **Clitoral Pumps**. So, what is clit pumping? These pumps are usually made of a cup, shaped like a cylinder, and a hand pump. The cup is placed over the entire outer clitoral area, and as you slowly squeeze the hand pump, blood will be drawn directly to the clitoris. The idea is to make the clitoris more full, firm and sensitive to the touch, which then leads to more powerful orgasms. Getting good blood flow to the clitoris is necessary for arousal, and more importantly for orgasm. The act of clit pumping can clear the way for anyone with a clitoris.

- **G-Spot Toys**. G-spot stimulation is unlike anything you are going to feel. It can feel out of this world. For some, it is the only way to consistently achieve orgasm. This is why G-spot vibrators have such a strong hold in the sexual wellness market. The Gräfenberg spot, more well-known as the G-spot, can be found on the anterior wall of the vaginal canal. When stimulated, it produces an intense sense of pleasure. A G-spot vibrator is specifically designed with an intended upward curve. This allows you to stimulate your G-spot quickly and easily. Most people indicate their G-Spot is located two to three inches inside their vagina. You should take two fingers and stimulate that area in a "come hither" finger motion, putting focus on the area more toward the front of your body.

- **Suction Toys**. Haven't heard about suction toys? Listen up, you won't want to miss this. The best of the best clit suckers are actually designed to mimic oral sex. These beauties are compact, whisper quiet, and promise intense, hands-free orgasms. Depending on the brand, each of these toys operate a bit differently. Most stimulate the clitoris through pulsation and air technology. Unlike a regular vibrator, you don't need to have direct contact. Many of these use gentle bursts of air to simulate kissing and licking.

Erotic Play

- **Handcuffs and Restraints**. The world of consensually restraining or being restrained for pleasure is vast. One need just do a quick google search and you could quickly become overwhelmed with the equipment alone. This realm of pleasure should always begin with a conversation with your partner. A concrete level of trust needs to be in play here. Understanding your partner's level of comfort here is vital. Once all of the boundaries are in place, it is time to experiment and have fun. Start slow with some silk wrap ties and once you are comfortable, you can explore leather cuffs, handcuffs, or hogtie cuffs. Do your research with your partner and have fun. Keep in mind, bondage type play doesn't have to conjure up images of dark dungeons, leather hoods, and chains. This is your story; do what makes you comfortable. If a sex room with all the tie down and sex benches is your thing, do it up right. If you are more at ease being tied up on your own bed, do that. The end goal is joy and heightened pleasure. Remember to use those safe words.

- **Nipple clamps.** A nipple clamp is intended to pinch small bits of your nipple flesh, essentially restricting blood flow to the nipple. Why would someone want to do this? Well, this creates a trifecta of pleasure+pain+numb=heightened sexual arousal. So, where does one begin? If you are a newbie to the world of clamps, it is best to start with an adjustable pair, that way, you are in control of the amount of pressure placed on the clamp. Every person varies in their desired amount of pressure, so having the ability to dial it up or down is a benefit. Why else do people enjoy a good nipple clamp?

  We all love good nipple stimulation, but there are times we wished we had a second pair of hands. With clamps, our nipples can be attended to, leaving our hands to do other stimulating work. One very important piece of advice to remember is if you are wearing the clamps and you are about to orgasm, timing is everything. If a nipple clamp is slightly uncomfortable before an orgasm, it will be very painful after.

Dr. Sadie Allison shares a tip about clamps. She says that "for some cis-men, nipple play is an extremely pleasurable and preferred type of stimulation. For others, they may have overlooked this erogenous zone altogether, so it's worth an introduction."(Hsieh & Varina, 2021)

Okay, so what are the tricks of the trade when it comes to nipple clamps? The last thing you should be doing is grabbing a pair of clamps and chomping down on your nipples. Preparing the area is a crucial step you don't want to mess with. Step one is to warm the temperature of the skin. We are aiming for a nice, long foreplay session here. Cup the breasts and massage the area, making sure not to miss the nipples, and slowly start licking and sucking on those nipples.

When you notice your partner is aroused, have them take a slow, deep breath while you clip the clamp onto the nipple. Ask them to slowly exhale. You will need to continue loving up on those breasts and nipples, as it may take a moment for the nipple to respond. Again, timing is everything. Pay attention to those cues, and when your partner is about to climax, remove the clamps. This is important because we need that blood to flow back to the nipples. In addition to that, the nipple stimulation releases oxytocin (also released during orgasms), so they are in for a double whammy. Nipple clamps come in a huge array of shapes and sizes, so do your research and have fun while you are exploring.

- **Hot Wax**. If you and your partner are looking to actually heat up the bedroom, this may be exactly what you are looking for. Wax play involves heating up wax and having it dripped on to your body by your partner, by yourself, or you doing the dripping on to the body of choice. The pleasurable sensation is all temperature related. Keep in mind here that you are playing with fire, literally, so safety first. Wax play for some is all about the pain for pleasure. Having the hot wax poured on them and feeling that momentary sting heightens their senses. For others, they get ramped up feeling the wax peeled off their naughty bits. Having the wax harden over their nipples, or yes, even the penis, but then the sensation of peeling that wax off sends them into ecstasy, toes curled and all. There are some steps you should follow to be prepared and be safe.

    - **Prepare your skin.** You should take some extra time to prepare your skin. Just grab your favorite lotion and give yourself a quick rub down. It makes getting the wax off so much easier and it prevents any irritations from the wax too. If you happen to have yourself a hairy partner, you may want to suggest shaving. Wax hardening in body hair is nothing short of a painful disaster; just trust me on this one.

- **Choose appropriate wax.** In the game of hot wax, not all candles are created equal. Do yourself a favor (and your partner) and don't grab that sparkly, pumpkin spice latte scented candle from your coffee table. Those particular candles get far too hot and are filled with extra additives. They are bound to irritate and aggravate your skin, after it burns you... I highly recommend an all-natural, organic soy candle. The scent is much lighter, and the wax temperature doesn't reach melt your skin off levels.

- **Safety check.** So, you have chosen the perfect candle, now what? Safety check is next, you want to be sure you have nothing flammable close to where the action is going to take place. Those fuzzy blankets or stuffed animals, drapery, or hairspray. Take a good look around and ask yourself, "what can catch fire here?" It is always wise to keep a fire extinguisher, or a bucket of water close at hand for those emergencies we don't foresee. Better safe than sorry.

- **Test.** The last thing you keep in mind before playing is pain. Always test the wax on the back of your hand before pouring. Your intention is never to hurt your partner, but accidents happen when we forget how long the candle has been burning. Remember to check in with those safe words and have fun. One last thought before leaving this item: If you want to add another layer, you can blindfold yourself to heighten the senses even more. Enjoy!

- **Bondage Kits**. If you are curious about dipping your teeny toe into the kink world of BDSM (bondage, discipline, dominance, submission, masochism), bondage kits are a good start. This level of sexual pleasure is all about your level of comfort. For those starting out, a beginner's kit is recommended. This allows you to test the waters, see what interests you and then you can expand based on what worked well. Handcuffs are a must; it just depends on the type you want, leather, silk, or padded. The choices are endless. An over the door sex swing, with a seat, offers versatility for positioning and bondage. Blindfolds are also needed, and the market has plenty to choose from. An ankle spreader bar that attaches to each ankle, prohibiting your partner from closing their legs. Great addition to your beginner kit. Sex pillow for positioning and comfort because some of these sessions can be long. Adjustable nipple clamps, because no two nipples are created equal. Your preferred tool for spanking, whether that be a paddle, crop, or just your hand. Last, bondage tape, as it is versatile and reusable. Great for keeping your submissive right where you need them. Keep in mind that BDSM is all about safety and consent. Keep those lines of communication open and those safe words handy.

Visual Play

- **Play Dress Up in Bed**. Dressing up in something naughty or nice is another way to spice things up in the bedroom. According to new research it could be one of the most effective when it comes to turning your partner on. A survey, commissioned by End of Tenancy London, found that 66% of Brits want their partner to dress up and 94.4% of those asked had tried it before (Meyerowitz, 2020).

    Though you can let your imagination run wild with just who, and how, you dress up as, the new research found that there was one outfit genre in particular that is sure to get your partner's heart pumping: the French maid. Yes, we know it might seem slightly clichéd, but it seems to do the trick, as one in five of the 1,451 participants asked preferred this outfit (Meyerowitz, 2020).

    On the flip side, figures of authority (think: police officer, nurse etc.) are also a big thumbs up in the bedroom; dressing up as a police officer was the fifth most popular outfit choice, tied with superheroes. So, if you've ever wanted to be She Hulk, now is your time. Remember; the key to making dress up work is feeling confident in what you're wearing, so choose an outfit that you feel good in.

- **The Use of Mirrors**. Mirrors can be a great way to enhance your sex life. Even if you don't use them all the time, it is good to switch things up a bit to increase sexual intimacy in your life. Some people are visual beings and very turned on when seeing their partner naked. During intercourse or other acts of foreplay, mirrors can help you be more stimulated with sexual desire. Some of us have a hard time staying mentally focused during lovemaking, seeing what is going on can really help. You can focus less on what you need to grab at the grocery store tomorrow and more on what is happening right in front of you. Using mirrors also allows a mental recall later. Having these images stored in your mind gives you something to visualize. Think in the middle of a Wednesday workday and flashes of your mirror scene pop in. You're welcome.

- **Sex games**. When was the last time you played a really great board game? Maybe you thought your days of game playing were over? Well, think again. There are some spicy R-rated games that you should not be missing out on. However, if you are sitting back wondering why on earth you should play a game about sex instead of just having sex, the answer is simple... foreplay! Sex games were invented to get you turned on, before you get it on. I personally am a big fan of the original games such as Twister, or Pictionary that manufacturers have put a sexy spin on. If you lose a turn, you are often asked to strip or perform a naughty task. Don't knock it until you try it, but this is a great way to bring sexy fun back into the bedroom.

Positioners

- **Sex pillows**. These have taken a bad rap for far too long. First marketed towards seniors who still wanted to shake the sheets, but had bad hips or deteriorating joints. However, people of all ages are starting to see the benefit these beauties can bring to everyone's sexual encounters. A sex pillow offers even more options because of the unique angles you are able to achieve. Discovering amazing angles for oral sex, for example, could be uncovered by one lifted thigh or buttock. These wondrous pillows allow you to explore these new angles, never before seen, all while being comfortable. No, these are not the same as just a regular pillow. A sex pillow is typically a much firmer pillow and it is angled like a ramp. They come in many shapes and sizes, so do your due diligence. So, why do people use them? One of the biggest reasons is deeper penetration. When you put the pillow under your hips, it allows a lift of your butt, allowing your partner to make a much deeper penetration. This is a real bonus if you have a partner with a smaller penis. Get yourself one of these pillows and experiment; the end results are bound to be glorious.

- **Kegels and Pelvic Floor.** Women have been dealing with painful intercourse for years and oftentimes, it can be traced back to weak pelvic floor muscles. Your pelvic muscles are like any other muscle in your body; they can become weak and lax, but with the proper exercise, they can become strong again. Your pelvic muscles run under the pelvis, and they play a huge role in sexual intercourse. Taking a workshop for pelvic floor exercises will teach you movements to help contract and relax this group of muscles. There have been studies brought to light recently that show women who exhibit sexual discomfort have noticed an incredible improvement in the quality of their sex life through pelvic floor exercises. More comfortable penetration and less pain during intercourse are also significantly reduced when engaging in regular pelvic floor therapy (Agnieszka Radzimińska et al., 2017).

The ultimate goal of pelvic floor therapy is to strengthen the pelvic floor, allowing it to become more flexible. In turn, affecting the way the pelvis maneuvers during sex, making it a less painful and a more pleasurable experience.

Kegels are also used to strengthen the pelvic floor muscles. The benefit to these particular exercises is the convenience factor, as they can be done anywhere, anytime. So, how does one do a Kegel you ask?

- First, you need to locate the right muscle group. To do this, force yourself to stop urination midstream. That feeling you get when forcing that flow to stop, those are the muscle groups you are targeting. Now that you know what area you are aiming for, you can do these exercises in any position. When you are first starting, you might find it easiest laying down.

- Now, let's get that technique down pat. To get the most out of your Kegels, I want you to imagine you are sitting on a pea, yes, a pea. Now tighten those pelvic muscles as if you're picking up that pea. Give this a try for five seconds, then relax for a count of three.

- Try doing this in a quiet space where you can focus. You will achieve the best results if you can focus on only those pelvic floor muscles. It will take time to master this, but be mindful that you are not flexing your core, or thighs. Remember to keep breathing nice and calm.

- It will do your pelvic floor a lot of good to repeat this three times a day. To maintain good strength, you should be aiming for a minimum of three sets of 10 repetitions a day. For additional support there are pelvic floor devices available.

Mood enhancers

- While the sexual wellness market is flooded with options to enhance your mood and increase libido, many are more comfortable with an all-natural option. There are plenty of options available to you, I have listed the three most popular below.
    - **Red ginseng.** Known to increase the libido of women traveling the path of menopause as well as improve erectile dysfunction in men.
    - **Saffron.** A warm, delicious spice derived from the Crocus sativus flower. It is known to improve sexual dysfunction for those taking antidepressants.

- **Maca.** A root vegetable and it is thought to enhance sex drive and fertility. You can find this in multiple forms, powders, liquids, extracts, and capsules. Studies have shown a significant improvement in erectile dysfunction when used over a 12-week duration (Beharry & Heinrich, 2018).

- **CBD Oils.** In the pleasure wellness world, CBD is making people stand up and take notice. It is a fabulous addition to your holistic sexual wellness repertoire. First, let's be sure everyone is aware of what CBD is. It is a non-psychoactive chemical compound found in both hemp and cannabis plants. CBD can provide benefits on many levels. People use it to reduce inflammation, lower pain, relieve muscle tension, and lower cortisol levels. For people with vaginas, CBD can do wonders. It adds heightened arousal, increased lubrication, and what I consider a huge benefit, it lowers pain for those who have painful intercourse. For those graced with a penis, you are not left out. CBD can increase blood flow, helping get those penises erect and stay harder, longer.

- **Pleasure Enhancement Supplements.** There is much debate surrounding the world of pleasure enhancement supplements. Do they work? Are they safe to use? They cover a large market of the pleasure business, but many do not hold up under medical scrutiny. They claim to bring back that libido that is lost, as well as sexual endurance. For example, a review was published in The Journal of Sexual Medicine in 2015, of the bestselling supplements for men's sexual health. They revealed next to no evidence to back any claims that they could improve any part of sexual performance (Harvard Health Publishing, 2022). While the general public feel they have a safety net with the Food and Drug Administration (FDA) in place, you should know they cover pharmaceuticals, not supplements. In the supplement world, you need to check your labels closely. They will often combine multiple ingredients and you need to know what you are ingesting. The two big ingredients you need to be mindful of are the following.

- **L-arginine.** This is in the amino acid family, and it supplies the raw material from which the body produces nitric oxide. This molecule promotes relaxation and opens up the blood vessels. This is a fundamental step in achieving an erection. "But putting that into a pill isn't proven to produce an erection," Dr. O'Leary says. He reiterated that a study of L-arginine's effect specifically examining heart attack survivors had to be halted due to the untimely death of six people taking the supplement (Harvard Health Publishing, 2022). Any person diagnosed with heart disease needs to consult with your doctor before considering this product.

- **Yohimbine.** This is derived from the bark of a tree native to the African continent. "It does promote penile blood flow, but you have no idea whether the supplement you're taking has too much or too little," warns Dr. O'Leary (Harvard

Health Publishing, 2022). There is another serious warning you need to be made aware of. Yohimbine can damage heart function and may trigger high blood pressure, insomnia, migraines, and night sweats.

When it comes right down to it, this is a buyer beware market. If you are going to try a supplement, I highly recommend talking to your doctor first.

Sexual Aftercare

So you've just done the dirty deed and you're feeling ecstatic with all those pleasurable sensations circling throughout your body. You've used your tongue, teeth, fingers, and your bits. You've sucked, licked, kissed, penetrated and rubbed. You've incorporated food, lube, handcuffs, a dildo, and a riding crop. You're sweaty, sticky and have knee and elbow burns from all your sexual frolicking. So, what happens next for you and your partner? Run to the shower? Condom removal? Strip the bed? Turn on Netflix? Sleep?

Sexual aftercare is an important part of sex and sexual wellness. Whether you are having some solo-pleasure time or with a partner, there are benefits to practicing sexual aftercare. We spend so much time seeking our happy ending and then once the mission has been accomplished, we often move on to doing other activities. But we need to spend as much time being mindful of our bodies after sex as we do before sex. Aftercare can mean many different aspects of taking care of our bodies after we have a sexual experience including physical and emotional care.

Just think, you've just spent what could be minutes to hours (think tantric) in a mental state of arousal and physical sensations. You need to 'come back to earth' and have a semblance of civility again after moaning and grunting. Many assume that aftercare is only necessary for those who choose to partake in BDSM activities, that may cause more intense and sometimes pain-centered sexual sessions. However sexual activity at any intensity can cause anyone to be left feeling physically and mentally impacted during your session. Sexual aftercare does in fact come from the BDSM community as a way to check-in on partners after a session. Many people can experience after sex dysphoria and injuries that need to be attended to. That being said, whether you are into kink or you keep it vanilla, having an aftercare plan has many benefits for you after sexual activity.

- **Prevents an emotional 'drop'.** After your sexual experience, you feel like a superhero with all the pleasure hormones like dopamine and oxytocin coursing through your body. However, once all the dust starts to settle inside your body, without taking a moment to be mindful about your experience with your partner, an emotional drop may occur. It's good to check in on each other after your experience to wind down like a feather rather than a led balloon.

- **Prevents Stress.** Sex (hopefully) brings out the inner wild animal in you. While you are in your state of arousal, your mind and body are focused on reaching your orgasm. You're much less concerned about your naked body, having a hookup, or trying a new sexual experience. However, once the deed is done, some people may experience anxiety, shame, or mixed emotions afterward. As I mentioned earlier, much of our formational thoughts around sex have been shaped by society, religion and our parents. For some, sexuality isn't a freeing experience right off the bat. Even as consenting adults, some find engaging in sexual activity as shameful. It's important for partners to ensure that the other is feeling safe and valued after your experience.

- **Provides safe space**. Additionally, there are some that may have suffered some form of sexual trauma in their past. Checking in on each other is an intervening way to support your partner to feel safe and secure with you during moments of sexual intimacy.

- **Provides opportunity for discussion**. Picking up the last point, sex can leave some feeling unsure of their performance and unsure about their experience. Prioritizing aftercare would allow for partners to take time out to honestly talk about their sexual experience, soon after it happens. Have you ever had a 'less than stellar' sexual experience? I have. I faked my way through it and said nothing about it afterwards. Not sure my partner cared about how my experience was either. By creating an open and safe space to discuss your experience in real time, both partners may be more likely to be honest about what was a hit and what was a miss in bed.

Aftercare Examples

Many of us already partake in some form of aftercare so these examples certainly will not surprise you. Its more so being intentional and mindful about looking after your sexual partner as a part of your intimacy. Here are the most common aftercare examples:

- **Clean up**. After the deed, spend some time cleaning up the bed, clothes and room. Wash up if you can, preferably together and may be groom each other if you want. Just warm water and mild soap on your sensitive skin, especially those thoroughly active parts. Also remember to clean up all of the sex toys you've used. Again, don't use any overly fragrant soaps, just a mild soap with warm water.

- **Sooth.** Depending on how intense your experience was, if there any sore or sensitive spots or burns, take time to put a cold cloth, cold compress or calming cream on your partner.

- **Refreshments.** After all the physical exertions and sweating, it's always good to rehydrate with some water and maybe a light snack. Feed each other and make sure you're both satisfied.

- **Calm it down**. Turn on soft lighting and use essential oil diffusers with lavender for better relaxation and calm and, of course, candles are always a nice touch.

- **Cuddling.** Yes, this can be a four-letter word to some but it's such an effective way to make your partner feel secure. In clean bedding cover, wrap around each other and spend some time giving gentle kisses or massages.

- **Watch TV.** Turn on one of your favorite shows that make you both laugh or you find super entertaining. Not many things feel better after a good orgasm than having a good laugh. So many good feelings inside your body. Savor them all.

- **Pillow talk.** No, it's not having a long-drawn-out discussion about where the relationship is going after having sex. Its more so talking about how the experience was and how you'd try something new next time.

- **Comfy clothes.** Wear nice, cooling and loose clothing and be comfortable if you plan to spend the night together. Avoid putting on any tight underwear on your sensitive skin.

- **Sleep.** This is more about being intentional to rest after your session of sexual expression and not just rolling over and snoring. After some or all of the other aftercare items are taken care of, be mindful to get a good night's sleep or a mid-day nap.

It's important to look at sexual aftercare as part of your sexual experience. It's not a chore or an obligation. It's to ensure that you and your partner are in a good headspace and feel mentally and physically whole after doing the deed. It can certainly lead to another session of getting it on if you're up to it. Picture talking about how good you felt, caressing any sore spots or gently bathing or showering each other and carefully massaging calming lotion on your skin. Does that sound like a chore to you because it sounds like round two or three to me.

CHAPTER 6: Prioritizing Your Mental Health for Better Sex

"I would rather cuddle then have sex. If you're good with grammar, you'll get it"
—**Unknown**

I know what you're thinking, *what does my mental health have to do with my sex life?* I am so glad you asked. Statistics pulled from the Canadian Mental Health Association (CMHA), shows us that 20% of us will deal with some form of mental illness during our lifetimes (Canadian Mental Health Association, 2021). So, that tells me that even if you personally aren't struggling with mental illness, someone you know, love, or are having sex with, could be.

Keeping that in mind, we have to remember that sex is not just a physical act. We, in fact, do spend a great deal "inside" our own head when it comes to sexual pleasure. It's crucial to remember that, our feelings and desires play a vital role in lighting our sexual fire, getting us heated up, and keeping us that way.

Mental health issues such as depression or anxiety disorders are not discussed enough when it comes to how they can impact arousal and mood. How often do we discuss how these issues make it almost impossible for the person to relax and truly enjoy the moment. Instead of feeling all the pleasurable things around them, their minds are filled with catastrophic thinking or dread. It can be hard as their partner to not take these moments personally, but try to understand how difficult it can be to crave sex or intimacy when you are struggling just to function.

Mental illness often hurts a person's self-esteem, which then makes them feel unworthy of any attention, but especially sexual attention.

Sexual Mindfulness

The importance of our brain when it comes to pleasure and sex is evident. What is sexual mindfulness and how can we use it to our advantage? The sexperts agree, your brain is the most valuable sex toy you own. It doesn't cost you a thing; you never have to charge it, and it is always readily available. It is all about learning to stay present, in the moment, and training yourself to not go on autopilot.

Sexual mindfulness is not just here to give your physical and mental health a boost—when you use it in the bedroom, it can heighten your pleasure and level of arousal. I am fascinated with some new research that has recently come to light. It is linking the part of your brain that pauses right before you have an orgasm to the same part that snoozes while you are meditating, or being mindful.

It can be so hard to stay in the mood, or even get in the mood when our brains are dragging us back to our daily lives, thinking 'did I put the garbage out?' or 'did I pay that cable bill?' This is a common occurrence with most of us, but there is great news. With some guided intention, not only can you stay focused, you can be sexually fulfilled.

Practice Making Mindfulness a Daily Habit

The old adage practice makes perfect rings true here. For sexual mindfulness, you are going to start by practicing being present in the daily tasks. For example, let's start with your morning shower. I want you to act like this is your first shower experience ever. Pay attention to all of your senses: Taste the tiny water droplets as they bounce off your lips, breathe in the scent of shampoo, lather up your hands and feel them slide across your skin.

For the entire day, I want you to be on high alert for each task you do. Something as simple as brushing your hair. Pay attention to how the bristles feel as they tickle your scalp. If you are doing some dishes after dinner, be mindful of the texture of bubbles across your skin and the running water cascading over you. The purpose of this, you ask? The more you practice, then each time your mind wanders during those times you want focus, you can recall these intimate sensations. You will be amazed at the recall of your own brain. The minute you are trying to focus on an intimate session with yourself or a partner, and your thoughts wander to the grocery aisle, just ask for a recall and you may get goosebumps thinking of the soapy shower.

Body Positivity

There are plenty of misconceptions swirling around the world of sex and pleasure, and body image doesn't escape this. Whether depicted on television, in the movies, or all over social media, we have painted a picture of beautiful humans having sex like rabbits. Their slim, chiseled bodies and their gleaming white teeth, this is the ideal picture that conjures up in our minds as the quintessential demographic who enjoys the most sex. This couldn't be further from the truth.

There is a direct link between body image and sex. How we feel in our own skin affects how we carry ourselves sexually. Any gender, body type or personality can have sky high self-esteem between those sheets. Research is showing us that those who feel good in their own skin, respect, and accept their bodies are more likely to be having great sex, according to a review of research that links our body image and sexual wellbeing (Gillen & Markey, 2018, p.191-197). If you're thinking that only the pretty people are having great sex, think again!

When we put all of this data together, we know that a better sex life isn't achieved by changing our body, it comes from changing how we *feel about* our body. When we get all up in our head about what the societal norm is and what the sexual expectations of us are, we shut down. Insecurity seeps in, sexual desire plummets, and we forget that the end goal was pleasure at all. This just does not work because confidence is one, if not *the* biggest aphrodisiac we have. Think about the last time you felt amazing. When you are in that headspace, you feel invincible. Like a naked superhero, ready to leap tall buildings, if you catch my drift.

The Modern Intimates Business

All I can say is, it is about time the intimate business is evolving. One of the last businesses to do so, they have a bit of catching up to do. Some newer brands like *Skims* blew the doors off this market by including everyone. Why, you might ask? Simple, every human that walks this earth loves to feel confident and sexy. Not just while they are flirting or tempting a mate, but also in everyday life. Can you recall the last time you walked into a meeting at work rocking the sexiest underwear set under your clothes? The last time you went to the grocery store holding your head high because you are wearing an article of clothing that makes you feel like a million bucks? Well, intimate apparel companies have been gearing their luxurious items to predominantly slender people for decades.

Along came social media and a slew of strong voices demanding space for more diverse and inclusive lingerie. It has been a beautiful thing to see, as billboards and advertisements began to bloom with visions of all skin tones and body shapes. This is normal; this is what humanity looks like. Its empowering to normalize average sized people in sexy clothing now. You no longer have to look as if you were starving yourself in order to buy pretty things.

There is a much larger and positive trickle-down effect we know is coming from all of this. How many of you, as young adolescents, would flip through ads and see those paper thin models, and think that was the standard to achieve? As impressionable youth, it was all we saw. Without knowing this was going to happen, society's expectations fueled the fire of eating disorders among many other mental health disorders, all in the hopes of becoming what society told us was beauty.

Imagine the change we are now creating. More of us now have the opportunity of seeing what real people look like as sexy. Happy, loving, beautiful, and accepting. This should have a positive effect on them; less pressure to starve themselves in order to fit into society.

The next time you want a little pick me up, hop online to any intimate supplier, or go out to one of their locations and see how much they have changed. Gift yourself something to light your inner pleasure beast or sex god. We all deserve to feel amazing, even if we are picking up dinner at the grocery store.

So, get out of your own head and practice those daily mindfulness techniques. Continue to build on your body image and self-esteem because the bigger they are, the better your sex life will be.

Sex Journaling

Most of us equate journaling to something we started in school to discuss what we did on the weekends, a way for our teachers to monitor our grammar and get to know us a bit better. As we bloomed into adults, some of us then took to journaling as a way to deal with childhood trauma or anxiety. It is a great way to track health, financial, or even travel goals.

Journaling has many benefits, but have you ever considered it as a way to improve your sex life? A sex journal is put in place to help you look back on your experiences, pleasures, techniques, and even fantasies. Below, I have compiled a list of some great reasons to start a sex journal of your own and tips on how to use one.

Helps Process Sexual Experiences

Journaling has been primarily used to help people reflect back on their thoughts and feelings. The main reason journaling is effective is because it "encourages expressive writing and helps people contextualize past emotional experiences," says sex therapist Lisa Hochberger. Let's be honest here, when we are in a state of passion, many things are happening at once. It can be a lot to process during that time, so giving yourself the time and space to journal about it is time for reflection. Not with a partner right now? Journaling is still quite effective if you are exploring your own body too. Reflecting on past sexual experiences or even some new techniques you want to explore are wonderful things to journal about. Sex lives can get complicated with many moving parts, so get out a journal and write; it is a great way to process.

You'll Gain an Understanding of Your Sex Life

Why do we do what we do in our sex lives? In the beginning, we are just figuring out how to have good sex, and not feeling so awkward being naked with another person. As we go along in life, it can become repetitive and just trying to achieve that orgasm. Now is the perfect time to slow things down. Journaling about our experiences provides that opportunity to become more aware of why we operate the way we do. What motivates and excites us, and seeing it all in black and white on paper, can be revealing.

If you have noticed slumps or a lack of drive, journaling can also help see patterns here, too. Tracking those ebb and flows may uncover things you never considered. You might find you are having more sex just before your period hits. Did you notice a pattern of heightened sexual arousal when your partner spanked you or tugged on your hair? Keeping track of these things in your journal can give you your own personal map to unlock what makes you tick.

Sex Therapy

As we have touched on earlier in this book, the stigma with mental health is slowly beginning to fade. We all either have a therapist, or know someone who does, and we need to continue on this forward path. So, what exactly is sex therapy and how can we make it more mainstream? Much like taking the stigma out of mental health, we need to continue to take the shame out of pleasure, sex, and all things self-love. Sex therapy is a great place to start.

People might be surprised to know that sex therapy has been around for decades. It is intended to help singles, or couples, learn how to live in the world of sexual wellness. You might also be shocked (or maybe not) that most people gather their sexual knowledge from social media, movies, or misguided google searches. Why? Because many are still uncomfortable talking about it. Sitting in front of a sexpert and discussing painful sex or the inability to achieve orgasm makes us feel abnormal, when, in fact, there are many with the same experience. If images of the film *Meet the Fockers* pops up in your head when you think of sex therapy, it's not that at all. You are not entering that office to discuss nakedness, or ways to improve your sex life.

People seek out a sex therapist for plenty of reasons. Here is a basic breakdown. When it comes to regular medicine, it is still locked in a treat one symptom at a time mentality. A patient comes in with a headache, we treat the headache and send them on their way. That same patient may return two or three times complaining the headache is still persisting, and the doctor then tries a few more approaches. If the approach would have been to treat the patient as a whole, a remedy would have been found much sooner. A quick intake from the patient regarding mental health, sleep, new food intake, etc., could give the doctor a clearer picture than just treating the head itself.

It works the same way with sex therapy. If someone is experiencing erectile dysfunction or ED and is frustrated, we could easily prescribe medication, but that same patient may return. They will still be frustrated because we are only treating the penis. Erectile dysfunction is caused by some medical issues such as high blood pressure or diabetes, but there are also links to depression and anxiety. As a sex therapist, it would be neglectful to not treat the mental health issues as well. Sessions to discuss any and all issues related to their expectations for pleasing others sexually, their body image, and anything else that can impede their erection would all come into play.

Sex therapy is an amazing treatment option for anyone having issues stemming from any of these sex concerns:

- having no sexual desire
- premature ejaculation
- erectile dysfunction
- difficulty being aroused
- menopause
- painful sex
- body image

- trouble having orgasms
- anxiety
- intimacy issues because of chronic pain, and
- conflicts with partners about sexual frequency or sexual activities.

Tantric Sex

What is tantric sex? In simple terms, you are intended to slow it all the way down. No more going at it like rabbits and hoping for the best. Slow down and enjoy every intense feeling, and most importantly, the build-up. Think of it in terms of the complete opposite of a two-pump jump or a quickie. Tantric is about experience, pleasure, and enjoyment while increasing intimacy.

Tantric is an ancient Hindu practice, and it has been in place for over 5,000 years. Tantric translates to "the weaving and expansion of energy" (Hutchings, 2022, p.1).

I know many are intimidated when they hear talk of tantric sex, like one must study for decades with a spiritual leader to achieve inner sexual greatness. I want to keep this all simple. If you look at a typical quickie like ordering pizza for dinner, we can compare tantric to dining at the most exclusive French restaurant where a jacket is required! You know the kind of place I mean, right? The food is prepared slowly; you can smell it wafting from the kitchen as it tickles your nose. The anticipation is intense as your stomach growls in anticipation. You sip on your cool, crisp wine, waiting for that delicious meal. It is set in front of you, and it is so visually stimulating, you don't touch it at first, you just want to drink in all of its gorgeous colors and textures. You bring the first bite to your lips, still wet from the wine, and slide it slowly in. Your jaw instantly tingles and goosebumps form on your neck. This is unlike anything you've ever tasted.

See what I did there? You can have pizza out of a box, or you can have an experience. Tantric experts believe, and teach, that if you extend the amount of effort and time you wait before intercourse, you are destined for higher and more intense bouts of ecstasy.

Trying out Tantric Sex

1. To begin, **lower the lighting** in an attempt to close out the rest of the world.

2. **Relax the body;** tantra's intention is to move energy through the body.

3. **Remove yourself from the bed:** We don't want any part of you getting tired, and this, being the place you sleep, makes you sleepy. We are retraining the brain to think, this bed is not only used for quickies and sleep.

4. **You need to be comfortable:** Lay down with your partner on a cozy blanket, but on the floor. You should slowly begin to touch one another, but keep in mind, your pace should be like this is the first time you are exploring their body.

5. **Experiment:** Try out a few different touches—barely touching, tickle, and then firmer. Your goal here is to arouse senses, getting close to the peak, but not to the top. Doing this exploring can prolong the act of sex and allow you to enjoy the pleasure for hours.

6. **Don't forget the breathing:** If your mind wanders, focus on your breathing. Think back to those journal entries you may have made, or recall those moments you used during meditation. Bring yourself back to the moment.

7. **Stick with it:** If you struggle to last 10 minutes, give it another try. Be gentle on yourself. Tantric sex takes time to master, but look at the fun you are having while you learn. Many of us are conditioned to sex in a Western way—we believe sex to run in a linear fashion with a beginning, middle and a grand ending. Just be patient, it will come.

Somatic Sex Education

Considered controversial to some, this form of sex therapy has some legal eagles up in arms.

Somatic sex education (SSE) is a form of sex therapy, which people engage in alone or they can choose to incorporate their partner. The sessions will always begin with talk therapy. Discussing the issues that have brought them to SSE, how long it has been going on, and any other information the therapist may deem helpful. That is exactly where this form of therapy stops resembling therapy at all.

From that point on SSE begins to direct the attention to how the client feels in their body. Now, wait for it because this is the controversial part. There are times the client may remove their clothing to be more comfortable.

There can also be occurrences of the therapist discussing the option of sexological bodywork. This would include the therapist physically touching the clients' genitals. Now, you may be asking yourself what kind of session this is, but this is done to show a client ways to eliminate painful intercourse, how to be mindful and present during sexual pleasure moments, or even how to achieve orgasm. Still not onboard? They also claim there is no easy way to describe this in a traditional sense, so feeling it just makes sense.

Some SSE therapists have compared this to how difficult it can be to learn to drive, but once you have someone beside you showing you what to do, it takes no time at all before you are a pro.

These therapists make it clear that their purpose is to educate and heal. Once the client identifies their reason for seeking out treatment, a plan is put in place. Whether they are there to begin enjoying sex again after childbirth, or after reassignment surgery, SSE therapists want to help.

The law surrounding this form of therapy is very clear. In Canada, it is illegal to exchange money for any form of sexual touch. There is no clear definition for the role as an

SSE therapist. You take money and touch in a sexual manner.

When we lay all our cards on the table, this form of therapy isn't going to be for everybody. The intention is to help get you connected with your own body, and to teach you what feels right for you. If you, as a consenting adult, want to invest in this, that should be your decision. It is a very new form of therapy, but I do believe it is one that may gain traction. Where does one go to learn form or technique? How do we know where to begin sometimes, especially if we have blocked trauma or years of shame? Baby steps for now, but I highly recommend keeping an eye on this one.

For many, their sexual journey hasn't been paved with unlimited orgasms, paths of rose petals, and stories of fantasy. Instead, they may have had to deal with far too many negative sexual experiences.

Mental health and sex do go hand in hand. We have covered plenty of ways throughout this chapter on how they link up. Using even one of these tools can help you maneuver those waters and increase your sexual liberation, pleasure and wellness. Feel free to use a few of them together once you are comfortable.

CHAPTER 7: Exciting Your Sexual Connections

"Physics is like sex; sure, it may give some practical results, but that's not why we do it"
– **Richard Feynman**

There is much to be said about the comfort of being in a relationship. The familiar connection you establish with your partner goes a long way in building what can hopefully be described as a solid sexual relationship. We can also make an argument for today's dating scene and the convenience of casual sex. It is now easier than ever to find a willing and consensual partner to blow off steam with some enjoyable, pleasurable sex.

Unfortunately, a large part of the population is complacent with a dwindling and unsatisfied sex life once they become settled in a relationship or marriage. Life gets in the way, the daily stress of building families, our careers and even getting bored with each other. Follow along through the steps of dating, marriage, and sometimes divorce, as we find ways to keep sex an important part of your social life.

Dating

The way the majority of relationships will begin, the date. Whether you are set up on a blind date, met on an online dating app, or you've known each other for years, dating is the first step in all relationships. You will hear tales of glorious first dates; romance oozing from every corner and hopes of happily ever after. However, for every amazing first date, there are a dozen disastrous ones. We can all have a great laugh at these tales of horror, but experiencing even one can turn you off dating for years. The thought of having to put yourself out there again is draining. In order to find our pleasure partner, the love of our life, or just someone to have between the sheets, we have to get back on that horse. Giddy up!

The Excitement

It can be 2:00 a.m. and your finger is cramped, eyes are burning, yet you are still swiping right on Tinder, trying to find that perfect one. Maybe all you are searching for is the one who can make you quiver and moan. Either way, the excitement and anticipation of the new relationship is unlike any other. You have been talking for a week or so and have finally agreed to meet. Those decisions alone are exhausting. Friends will always tell you to keep it casual, family will tell you to meet in public, so you don't end up in a scary situation, and all you want is that earth shattering orgasm. Okay, first you want to be sure they are a decent, mentally stable human, and then... the orgasms. You get a great night's sleep the night before, make sure your best outfit is clean, you are showered, and all your naughty bits are prepped. The entire way to the meeting spot you feel like you are holding your breath. Over the course of the evening, during your conversations, you have felt a connection. You have shared wonderful conversations, mutual interests, and so much laughter. You both seem to have similar values; so, what more could you ask for? Oh right, that orgasm. We will have to see how that all works out.

The Reality

You arrive at the restaurant five minutes early, hoping your date is already there and you can make an entrance. You send a quick text letting them know you are on your way in. You let the host know which reservation you are, and quickly find out you are the first to arrive. You will soon find out you will be waiting 45 minutes for your date to show. Eventually, they arrive at this semi-formal restaurant in what can only be described as "what they rolled out of bed in." Okay, it is just clothing, we can move past that. As they rush in, with zero apology for their tardiness, you stand for a friendly hug, but they quickly sit. Alright, moving on, you graciously smile, letting them know you went ahead and ordered a drink and a small appetizer but didn't know what they would like to drink. You are met with a bit of a snarky attitude when you are informed, they don't drink and are not fond of people who do. Interesting plot twist but, nonetheless, you carry on. Over the next painstaking three hours, you are subjected to rants about politics, annoying people in the workplace, and all of the disastrous relationships they have been stuck in throughout their life. Not one inquiry about your life, and you are racking your brain for an excuse to bolt. The bill is placed on the table, and they jump from their seat, claiming they need to run because their Uber has arrived. Wait, what? Stiffed with a hefty bill due to your date's love of expensive appetizers, you chalk this up to a learning lesson and contemplate whether to just live with cats.

The Challenges

Research is showing us that almost half of people in the United States believe dating is significantly more difficult now than it was 10 years ago (Barrosso, 2020). Reasons they feel this way include heightened risk, both emotionally and physically, and technology, making it so much more difficult to meet people. The truth is dating has never been a totally straightforward endeavor however dating in the 21st-century comes with many complications especially regarding sex. There are so many societal expectations that you have to consider. In a modern age we try to not be bound by restrictive gender expectations or puritanical restrictions and just live freely. But there are broader impacts we have to be mindful of as well as other precautions. Some people want to date just to have sex and some people date with the intentions of a long-term relationship and marriage. Just know that when it comes to dating, everyone is in the same boat since we all have to put ourselves out there. Here are some of the most common considerations when it comes to dating and sex.

- **Confidence.** Dating is nerve-wracking for most people. You put on your best outfit, smell nice and look nice but your palms are sweaty and your mouth is dry when you arrive at the café where you're supposed to meet your date. Why? Because you want to put the best version of yourself forward when you meet someone new. You want to be charming and mysterious, smart and sexy all at the same time. But what happens when the date progresses to intimacy and sex? Will you be as confident knowing your clothes are going to be off with that perfect stranger? Confidence in yourself is so important and absolutely sexy too. Prepare yourself for your date and be mentally and physically ready for someone else to see you naked. Remember the grooming techniques we went over earlier. Be prepared.

- **Timing.** Should you have sex on the first date? On the third date? 90 days? Wait for a commitment? Deciding on when to have sex with a person you've started to date can be confusing. If you both are just looking for a casual sexual relationship then just make sure you are taking the proper precautions and respecting each other's sexual boundaries. Sex with someone new is fun and exciting and can teach you things that you didn't know before. If both partners don't have any expectations of a long term commitment then emotions don't have to get in the way of having some fun. That said just be sure that both partners are realistic about having a purely physical engagement. For some, good sexual compatibility may lead to an emotional attachment and create different expectations over time. Be honest with yourself and your partner about your expectations to avoid any undue emotional stress, confusion and heartache.

- **Catching feelings.** You had sex on a date. Although you initially thought all you wanted was sex from this person you really find them cool and intriguing and want to be with them for more than sex. For many that are looking for a deeper connection choosing to have sex too early can conjure up deeper emotional feelings that might not be there for you with your partner. This imbalance of emotions and feelings could add undue pressure on a relationship that can cause your partner to head for the hills. If you know that you might be one to catch feelings after having sex with someone you might want to hold off on physically engaging too soon. Self-awareness is very important here.

- **Double-standards.** Even in the 21st Century, women are still judged for wanting to freely express their sexuality. Although a woman can have sex with whomever she wants to there could still be societal blow back on her by labeling her as a slut or easy. While on the other hand, men don't have these societal pressures on them. It seems very archaic but many of these diverging perceptions still exist. The way I see it is, if society is going to brand someone as sexually loose, then what does their gender have to do with it? Answer, it doesn't.

- **Safety.** Whether you are casually dating or dating someone with intentions for something longer-term being safe and feeling safe is paramount. Going home with someone is a risk. A good looking and sexy stranger is still a stranger. The bare truth is that being naked in a stranger's home leaves you quite vulnerable and can put your safety at risk. Always make sure that someone knows where you are and who you're with. Insert eye-roll emoji. I know, I know how this sounds. If you have no intention of doing this that's fine. But hopefully you get the point. Acts of sexual violence are still prevalent around the world. Furthermore, over the past several years there has been an increase in the act of stealthing. Stealthing is the act of purposefully removing a condom during sexual intercourse without consent from a sexual partner. Many countries within the last few years have come to identify this act as a form of sexual violence. Pleasure is fantastic but nothing feels better than being safe.

- **Friends with Benefits.** Although self-pleasure is great, sometimes we have the desire to be sexually intimate with a partner. Dating can definitely scratch that itch but what if you're tired of meeting new people that you don't connect with or just aren't into. Many people have come to find that hooking up with an ex or a friend takes the edge off sexually. Hence, the term benefits. You don't have to deal with the awkward getting to know someone new on a date and there are no expectations for the relationship. It's just important for each partner to understand and agree that you'll remain just friends after the beneficial deed is done. In other words, the longer-term benefit is still having someone in your life as a trusted friend without the romantic attachments and expectations.

- **Polyamory.** Polyamory or also known as Ethical Non-Monogamy is having a romantic relationship with more than one person at the same time. Polyamorous relationships are certainly not new however with the growth and popularity of dating apps, polyamory has become more popular or mainstream as more people are exposed to the idea. Plural relationships have to be consensual and everyone aware of each person involved. As a consenting partner, you should be able to set your own boundaries for this type of relationship to work and be healthy. And as with all relationship's communication is absolutely essential.

Relationships and Marriage

If your dating life turns into something serious and a committed relationship ensues, then your next stage could be a long-term relationship or marriage. No two marriages are created equal. Social media has brought a new level of interpretation as pictures are splashed all over, depicting what perfection and relationships goals should be. What we need to remember is, a snapshot in time does not necessarily reflect the truth of a relationship.

The Excitement

Any new relationship is filled with the excitement of newness. Whether you dated for years or months before deciding to get married, that engagement breathes new life into the relationship. If you are in a long-term relationship, maybe you have both decided marriage isn't in the cards for you, but cohabitating is, and your next step is finding a place to move in together. These are all new and exciting steps in your journey together. The posts go up on social media for the world to see. "Jordyn is engaged to Ryder," the headline splashes across the screen, and the likes, hearts, and comments flood your inbox. You giggle with excitement as you respond to them all, posting pictures of the ring and answering questions about when the big day is. If you are in a long-term relationship and have decided to move in together, you might be posting photos of a sold sign on the front lawn of your new home together. Skipping through IKEA, picking out matching towels and new bedsheets, this is pure happiness.

All things new will always breathe excitement and joy into us. Cuddling together and planning out the future is the reason to flood our systems with all those feel-good hormones. If you are in the planning stages of marriage, there are plenty of celebrations leading up to the big day. For some families and cultures, these are massive, and you are surrounded by love and support. In other instances, you may be planning an intimate destination wedding for just the two of you. Booking those tickets and anticipating the vacation is enough to peel off your clothes and practice that sex on the beach you can't wait to explore. All of the feel-good hormones will be ravaging your body through all of these stages. Don't be surprised if your sex life takes a huge spike throughout all of these stages. The dopamine will be high and so will your sex drive. The romance of it all can have you looking at your partner with refreshed love and admiration. Keeping your hands, mouth, or any part of your body off of them may prove difficult.

The Reality

Counsellors often see couples experiencing challenges within the first 9 to 12 months after getting married. The next spike is usually seen around the five-year mark.

Let's begin with the wedding day itself. So many long and exhaustive hours can go into these events. I refer to them as events because some of them wind up becoming larger than life. What is meant to be a union of love between two people can explode into a show for all to see. Invitations can arrive at your door that resemble a hand-carved box, and upon opening them, a dove or butterfly floats to the sky. Hundreds of people arrive, some the couple haven't seen or communicated with for years. Flowers and decor, meals, music, not one, but multiple photographers, all costing more than most pay for a car. In all of this, the magic of the love that brought you both together is lost. Now, it is all about the stress. Will this all come together? Can we afford it?

At the end of this spectacle, you head to your wedding night venue. What loving couple doesn't want to get busy on their wedding night, right? A not so scientific poll was conducted on Twitter, and the results are in—24% reported having sex on their actual wedding night, but a resounding 62% said no way, they were too tired (Stewart, 2021).

This statistic doesn't surprise me in the least. Wedding days are exhausting and long, typically beginning earlier than your normal workday and not winding down until the wee hours. Who wouldn't want to get out of those fancy clothes, finally get something to eat, and get some sleep? Don't be too hard on yourselves here and set some realistic expectations. Allow yourselves some time to rest and refuel; by doing this, you are guaranteed a far more enjoyable sexual experience than if you throw yourselves at each other exhausted.

Okay, so you're all married up, or living together. The number one reason couples begin experiencing problems is communication. You believe the other partner should have super powers and read your mind. It typically starts off beautifully, flowers for no reason, a surprise dinner reservation or breakfast in bed. Then life happens, and if you don't communicate what is bothering you, your sex life can start to fall apart quickly.

Oftentimes, before the wedding or the moving in together, your sex life is hot and frequent. You were younger, and in all honesty, you were still trying to impress one another. We have been conditioned to believe that the trial period is when you have to hook them, pull out all the stops, and make sure you sell all your best qualities. During that entire phase, sex is happening constantly. It's happening in crazy places, and you are comfortable enough with one another to experiment.

Now, routines are setting in and time may be a bit scarcer. You may be planning a family and as you get a bit older, you will get tired!

The Challenges

Okay, let's break down the challenges you will inevitably face during marriage or long-term relationships and offer some solid solutions. I think it is important that we all understand the relevance of sex in any relationship. It is important. It is very important. It helps us stay connected to the person we love and care for. Learning ways to keep that connection intact will be crucial in saving your relationship.

Issues under the sheets can and will end a long-term relationship or marriage if they are ignored. Sometimes you will face physical issues like chronic pain, surgeries or circulatory issues that cause issues with sexual function. We often have to deal with emotional issues as a couple, such as depression, anxiety, or anger issues. All of these can be dealt with in therapy, but being aware of them and being willing to fix or deal with them will go a long way in saving your marriage.

Common Sexual Problems in Marriage

- **A Sexless Marriage.** A marriage without sex won't survive. As I mentioned above, that physical connection is necessary. You may be shocked (or maybe not) that roughly 15% of married couples operate with a sexless marriage (Collaborative Divorce Texas, n.d.) There is a portion of these couples that decide staying together for young children or finances is important and sex is not. It isn't too often this arrangement lasts long. One partner is usually comfortable with it, while the other is not. Divorce is typically right around the corner.

- **Withholding Sex for Control.** The average North American couple in a committed relationship is having sex roughly eight times each month. That sounds fantastic, doesn't it? The issue is, in some of these cases, it is just one partner controlling the narrative. Placing demands on when, where and how sex will take place and even withholding sex as a form of control. This is never going to end well, because as adults, nobody wants to feel controlled. Withholding sex in an attempt to punish the person you love will end your relationship. Nobody wants to feel rejected, and you are bound to create feelings of anger and resentment within your union.

- **Too Busy for Sex.** This one is a popular one, shared by many. "My partner thinks I am a superhero, I am taking care of two kids and working, I am too tired to get naked and have sex!" On the other hand some don't speak of it at all because they are expected to perform under all conditions, it is their duty. This all boils down to priorities, and if you claim you are too busy for sex, your priorities are off. If you have invested in self-help books, scented candles, or downloaded any apps to help you with finding more me time, then you clearly know the importance of putting you first. Sex should be on that list. We already know all of the amazing benefits it brings to you both mentally and physically, so why have you stopped incorporating it into your life now?

  For most, this is nothing short of finding the right work/life balance. We are so busy pleasing everyone else around us, the boss, the co-workers and the children, that we leave ourselves and our partner at the bottom of the list. If you want this marriage or long-term relationship to succeed, flip that list. You need to be number one, and your sex life needs to be at the top. Bring back those orgasms and sexual pleasure and watch how much stress melts away from your life.

- **Pornography**. Watching porn together is hot and can lead to some incredible sex. It can become a problem if one partner is substituting porn for actual sexual pleasure with their partner. There are times that pornography can become a legitimate addiction and when this happens, there is no longer a connection between the couple. An intervention needs to take place here with therapy. Don't shame your partner, just try to be as supportive as you can and help to find a reputable sex therapist.

- **Cheating on Your Spouse.** There is no sugar coating this subject. The trust that is built between couples should be paramount. Cheating on your partner can end your relationship or marriage. It causes severe personal pain and shatters any and all trust that was established. That trust may or may not be able to be rebuilt. Some couples view this as a wakeup call and immerse themselves in therapy; while others can never move past the betrayal.

You should be mindful of signs of sexual issues within your marriage or relationship. If you notice them, and choose to ignore them, you may be creating a world of unhappiness and no sexual pleasure, and that sounds like no fun at all. Remember, communication is key; try taking a positive approach here and have those tough conversations. Talk about sex and why it should be important and at the top of your list. Be sure each of you are able to talk about what you need and what you want. Each of your emotional and physical needs should be satisfied within your relationship. Doing something about it may save you from heading to divorce court.

Keeping Sex Hot

When life gets busy and you find yourself surrounded by the stress of work or raising children, it can be hard to keep sex fresh and exciting. Don't feel you are alone in this; it happens to us all. We go to bed this sexy vixen, clothed in red leather, tying our partner up, and we wake up with pajamas covered in baby vomit, having no idea where our sexy panties disappeared to. Life is all about ebb and flow, discovering and rediscovering who we are. There are some great ways to keep things exciting and fresh during the transitional times of your relationship. Here are a few to get you started:

- **Sex goals.** We all know the importance of setting goals for ourselves to aspire to. Financial goals, fitness goals career goals. There are so many books, apps, and businesses out there to help us become the best versions of ourselves. Well why don't we add sex goals to that list. Great, regular sex in your relationship may even help position you to reach your other goals outside of the bedroom with a clearer mind. Check out these ideas:

    o **Position of the week.** Create a 52 week calendar with a new position every week to try out. You'll have fun even researching which positions to add to your calendar. If you can't find enough positions that will be suitable for you, make variations of the ones you find really pleasurable.

    o **Location, location, location.** Make a list of fun and exciting and maybe even risky places to smash with your partner. Think backyard, balcony, to abandoned lot, early morning on a beach, random hotels. There are plenty of places. Get creative.

- **Get it in, first thing.** It's true, if you're not being woken up by kids, you're already thinking of having to deal with your annoying micromanaging boss at work. But the truth is, sex in the morning sets your day off right. I'm not looking for a long sensual love making session, this is a 'quickie for breakie' kind of goal just to help you take the edge off to start your day. Even if it's a tug-tug, rub and tug or rub-rub situation, get it in first thing.

- **Creative writing.** Each of you write a dirty story. Doesn't matter the length. Just enough to share some of your sensual thoughts with your partner. Read your story to your partner with dimmed lights and candles.

- **Get naked, everywhere.** Become exhibitionists in your home with your partner. On a lazy weekend don't make any plans except to be home doing random things, while naked. Cooking, cleaning, reading, cuddling, watching tv. Make sure there is lots of touching, grazing, kissing, caressing and fondling throughout the day.

- **Take a sex lesson.** Take a course on how to improve your sexual performance. Regardless of how great you think you are in bed, we can always learn more. Taking a course together can really help you learn more about what your partner wants and expose you each to new things to spice it up.

- **Prioritize kissing.** Sometimes we just want to get to the happy ending, but kissing is a foundational element of sexual intimacy. Remember how much you kissed when you first started dating, it probably felt like hours on end. But for some, overtime, long luscious kisses devolve into quick pecks here and there. Prioritizing kissing can be a fun and easy way to bring your sexy back to each other.

- **Become Body Cheerleaders.** Confidence is sexy. So what better way to feel sexy and get each other in the mood than to tell each other how amazingly sexy you both are. Make a goal to randomly, text how much you love their ass in that pair of jeans, or that sweater. Leave a private sticky note in their laptop bag telling them how much that black dress and heals outfit made it difficult to contain your excitement. Put a note on the bathroom mirror saying how they have aged like fine wine and you can't wait to be naked with them later. Now, build on this.

- **Pleasure mapping.** Sometimes you just have to be clear about what you want, what feels good and what doesn't. With your partner, draw or print out a body frame that best represents each of you. From here, be as descriptive as you need to be in writing down or coloring which body parts provide the most pleasure and what your partner needs to do to make you get off. Use markers, have a color code, descriptive words like 'much more licking here', 'clockwise circles there, 'much less pressure at the tip', 'bite more, bite harder outside'. Got it? Map it out to suit your pleasure needs.

- o **Let the song say it.** Sometimes songs say it all for us. That's why songwriters get paid the big bucks. Words matter and there are some sexy songs out there. Find the songs you like or have lyrics that really get you in the mood or celebrate your partner. Send them the link to the song so they can hear it and a quick note of why you sent that song. For inspiration, these are some popular and classic sexy songs.

    - 'You make me feel like a natural woman'
    - 'I'm so into you'
    - 'I want to lick you up and down, till you say stop'
    - 'All I think of lately, is how to get you underneath me'
    - 'Let's get it on'
    - 'Your sex takes me to paradise'
    - 'You're so sweet, so tight, I won't bite unless you like'

- o **Have a Sex-cation.** Plan a vacation to just get your freak-on. Only you and your boo. No friends, no kids. Just a few days away to shag. Bring your sex toys, bring your massage oil, bring sexy outfits, bring all you have in your sexual toolbox. Plan to plug out of all things external stimulation and plug into each other.

Maybe annually, bi-annually, quarterly, depending on your schedule. Could be a long weekend or a week doesn't matter, just make it happen.

- **Prioritize orgasms.** Not all of us easily have orgasms. If this is you, make a priority to working with your partner to communicate what brings you into orgasmic ecstasy. Be honest with each other so you can know how to best please each other.

- **Build a sex room.** Okay, this might be more of a sex bucket list entry for most but hear me out because it doesn't have to be the locked, 'red room of pain' from the movies. Depending on your living situation, you might be able to make portable sex apparatuses to suit your sexual needs. Think putting a sex sling on a door frame, red silk sheets on your bed, and dark curtains over your regular window coverings, a lockable chest or fire proof case for your feathers and handcuffs. Have a designated sex chair, or bench. You can customize your sex room anyway you want. And when you're ready to play, (meaning no one else is home) your regular bedroom is now a sex room.

I hope this list of sex goals can get you at least thinking about fun and exciting ways to enhance your sex life that you can aspire to and achieve. But here are some other reinforcements to keep things fresh and frisky in bed.

- **Dirty Talk.** Sex and passion happen between the body and the mind. Yes, your body is exhausted, and you may not have one ounce of energy to engage in a round of sex, but I bet you can still talk. So why not start there. Remember to get creative here, scribble some on the bathroom mirror, little notes in their lunch, or on the dashboard of their car. This is all about build up and here are a few to get you started.

    - "I want to explore all of your body with my wet mouth."

    - "The minute I lay my eyes on you, I am going to slowly undress you and pleasure you for hours."

    - "I need you to come over. I have a stiff drink and a stiffer problem only you can fix."

    - "Happy sexaversary, ready to celebrate with some new lube?"

    - "My flashbacks of last night are so hot I get wet with each visual."

    - "Every time I think of you today, my nipples get hard."

    - "Get that ass in my bed."

    - "I want to tease you until your thighs are quivering."

    - "Have you ever had sex until you are dehydrated? Me neither, wanna try?"

- "Once we leave this party, my panties will be falling off in the car."

- "I want to just use my tongue to explore all the places that make you moan."

- "Tonight, my goal is only pleasing you."

- "Tonight, you get a full body massage, I'll lube up all my favorite spots."

- "I'm eating light tonight... you're my dessert."

Okay, they may be a bit cheesy but you can write your own up based on your sex language with your partner. Now, imagine your partner's reaction to finding these hot messages scrolled across their phone.

- **Keep it sweet and light.** Food foreplay should be considered the appetizer, with sex as the delicious meal. Keeping this in mind, enjoy the spicy food for that dinner plate and engage in all the delicious sweetness for appetizers. If your house engages in all organic and no sugar, no worries. Bring that amazing plate of fresh fruit, think plump cherries, juicy mango, or ripe strawberries into the bedroom. Do you love all things candy? Why not make your body its very own sundae? You are the ice cream and offer up all the chocolate sauce, marshmallow spread, and sprinkles to top you. Feeding each other can be so hot, especially if your bodies are the plates. Imagine eating fruit salad off a breast, or licking chocolate sauce off a hard penis. A word of caution here, portion is everything. We can get excited with all of the options, but if you overindulge, you may feel bloated and too full to enjoy the final curtain call. There is nothing worse than being so horny you want to finish, and being nauseated at the same time.

- **Use all your senses.** Be sure to use foods that not only feel amazing on the skin but smell fabulous. To keep things hot, try foods you can heat up, like chocolate or honey. Flip the script and cool things down as well. Bring in some frozen grapes, ice, or even popsicles.

    Nipples love the stimulation of hot and cold. Watch as your partner moans and their back arches as you slide different temperatures over their skin. Don't ignore all the other erogenous zones, like the earlobes and the back of the neck. Remember, you also have hands that can explore their genitals (where the food isn't allowed) while playing with the food.

- **Sexting.** Sex plus texting equals sexting, and can spice up any relationship. This is one that you can adapt quickly and easily for even the most exhausted couples. There is no added expense or time. We are all on our phones multiple times throughout the day now, so putting in an intentional sext to your partner is feasible. Incorporate some of those dirty talk prompts from above into your sexting realm and watch your sexy time grow and flourish. Try something as easy as, "Hey babe, can you grab milk on your way home? Can't wait to be naked in bed with you and feel your rock hard wood against my thigh. See you soon!"

    While most believe sexting to be more for those newly dating or trying to be overly flirty, this isn't actually the case at all. Research is revealing to us that those of us in marriages or long-term relationships, who followed their sexy texts with a hot sexy photo reported having an increase in sexual activity of 35% and a rekindled emotional connection with their partner (Drouin et al., 2017).

- **Sex Playlist.** How many of you have playlists made for running, working out, or just to relieve stress when you are trying to sleep? Have you considered making a sex playlist? Music is a wonderful tool for helping us relax and putting us in particular moods. Think of all the great ways music enhances your life. If you are trying to enhance your sex life, bring music into the picture. Spend some time researching some of your favorite mood music and don't forget to keep your partner in mind here. Do you both have "a song" from your wedding or your first date? Romantic gestures go far in the sex department, but be sure to add those ballads that get your motor running as well.

  > The bonus to music, it can help drown out those loud moans and screams. If you are a parent, really letting loose becomes an issue when you just got the baby to sleep, or your teen is in the next room. Put that playlist to work, relax and let yourself run wild.

- **Send a Meeting Request.** Over the last few years, we have all been bombarded with Zoom meeting requests. The dreaded lengthy virtual work meeting, dressed professionally from the waist up, trying to keep the kids quiet, all so very stressful. I am suggesting we change this dynamic. How about you send your partner a meeting request? Will they be confused? Absolutely, but this is all part of the fun. Be sure you include in the instructions that the meeting is mandatory, and they should be in a private setting. Won't they be surprised when the meeting starts, and you are dressed (or half dressed) in sexy office attire? Role-play this up for an added sexy level. Be their boss doing a random evaluation while showing plenty of cleavage, or your penis on the desk. Want to bump it up a notch? Be completely naked when that meeting opens. Can you even imagine how excited your partner will be to get home that evening? You are welcome.

- **Sexual Fantasies.** We all have sexual fantasies, and they vary drastically from one person to the next. The key to exploring these with a long-term partner is trust and support. We need to offer a safe space for these conversations so our partner feels they can communicate these to us without ever feeling shame. I always like to suggest having a sex fantasy date night. This may not be what you think it is. You need to make a reservation for a nice place to eat. If this isn't in the budget or babysitters are hard to come by, prepare a nice meal at home, and get dressed up. The entire purpose is a relaxing meal and a lot of communication. As mentioned earlier, our brain plays a big part in our sexual pleasure. This entire date should be about safely discussing any and all fantasies we may have been thinking about or wanting to explore. If you want to have one date night for the first partner to discuss their own fantasies, and the next date will be for the next partner.

Listen for the reason of truly hearing your partner. Do your best to not respond in shock or horror. If something catches you truly by surprise, just take a small breath and ask questions. It is often just the lack of knowledge that has us confused or surprised. You may be pleasantly surprised to find how turned on you both become by listening to one another's fantasies. Once you have laid them all out, it is time to make a plan of action. This is always the fun part. Encouraging and supporting these will bring you both that much closer, but offering to fulfill these (whichever ones you are comfortable with) shows your partner your ability to hear them and support them.

- **Get Off the Bed.** Sex on the bed is as common as butter on toast. But it doesn't have to be. When you find yourselves in a sexual rut, this is one of the simplest and quickest ways to spice it up. Again, no extra added cost or time is needed here. When you are just starting out, and if you have a house full of children, you can still stick to your bedroom, if that is where you are most comfortable. Lay some nice smooth, silky sheets on the floor, of fluffy blankets. You will instantly be amazed at the new angles available to you off the bed. Have some different seating in your bedroom, utilize that as well. Next, ship the little ones off to the grandparents for the night and re-explore your entire home. Back to that shower sex you once enjoyed. Try sex on the stairs; those angles will bring you pleasure you may not have had before. Do you have a kitchen island? It will bring you to perfect heights, perfect for oral, and food or temperature play. Just be sure to sterilize once you are done.

Taking things outside the house is adventurous and makes some couples immediately ramped up just planning it. Just be sure you are safe and stay away from private property. Having to call family or friends for bail money is never pleasant.

- **Role-Play.** I am going to combine role-play and date night together here. Planning date nights can become cumbersome when you are busy and exhausted. Who is going to plan it; where are we going to go, and do we have the resources? Bringing in the element of role-playing may just be the added excitement you need. Why not send your partner a text letting them know that you have made reservations and would like them to meet you at a certain destination at a set time? Let them know what you will be wearing, and that you want to role-play. You've never met, you are a married woman, and they should attempt to pick you up. You are going to fulfill your fantasy of being flirted with by a dark haired Adonis. Really get into character with this. They invite you back to their room in the hotel, and who knows, elevator sex just might be the end result.

- **Intimacy Coaching.** This is something relatively new in the area of couples. If one, or both of you in the relationship, struggle with intimate forms of touching, an intimacy coach would be perfect.

An intimacy coach is a professional who aims to assist you in feeling safer and more at ease when being intimate with a partner. While most of us have no issues with this because we grew up in homes being nurtured, hugged, and loved, some did not. There are those who grew up with no physical connections or traumatic experiences and are now very uncomfortable with it.

The job of the intimacy coach is to help show you how to feel safe. We know physical intimacy, closeness and touching are all vital in relationships and marriage, so engaging with this professional can only be an added benefit for you.

- **Sex Workshops.** Looking for something to do together or alone, sex workshops are educational, informative and a lot of fun. They are intended to educate us in all things sex. From toys, to fantasies, and everything in between. You can select the exact topic you want more education on, find the date that works best for you and your partner and make a night out of it. Sitting through these with your partner will most certainly get those juices flowing. Some of the classes are listed below to give you a better idea.

    - how to improve your blow job
    - the basics of BDSM
    - all you want to know about handcuffs
    - sex toys and why you need them
    - lube and why you need it, and
    - how to make role-play hot.

These are just the tip of the iceberg, but now you can see why attending one may end in orgasms!

- **Sex Games.** The sexual wellness world is filled with sex games, some intended for groups and others for couples. You will want to do your research to discover which ones are meant for you both. These can bring about bouts of hilarious laughter and also heightened pleasure. They offer journeys of discovery and educational points as well.

We like sex games in this instance because we are trying to spice things up and break out of routine, and what better way to re-engage in playfulness than with a game? Mind you, these games may require a bit more planning than some of the other suggestions, but it will be worth it in the end.

The first and most important benefit of sex games is that you are more inclined to try something new when it is framed in a game setting. When our relationships get stale or comfortable, everything becomes very predictable. Bringing games into the mix adds that layer of surprise and excitement.

There are actually hundreds, and that is not an exaggeration, of sex games on the market. Spend some time figuring out what might interest you and lock that bedroom door!

- **Kamasutra Yoga.** The ancient Sanskrit text popular for its guidance on intimacy, sexual health and eroticism can be an amazing tool for any couple looking to enhance their sex lives. There are many classes available that focus on yoga poses to promote sexual intimacy between partners. If you're not shy and looking for a fun way to loosen up while getting your sexual sparkle on, give it a try.

- **Food.** We all love food, and it is so easily accessible in your home. No excuses as to why you can't incorporate it quickly and easily! The obvious question is, how would one begin using food to spice up your sex life? Before you begin, be sure to use foods that won't trigger an allergic reaction. Follow the tips listed for the best possible outcome when introducing food into your sex life.

  > Just beware, keep food out of the sex holes. I know you may have seen some porn flicks where this is not the case. They get paid good money for that; you do not. Genitals and food don't mix. Think skin irritants, matted pubic hair, and a real risk for infection. Now, if you grab the ice cube tray, you can explore any and all places with no worries. If you grabbed the ooey-gooey chocolate syrup or any other food element, you are best to stay above the waist.

- **Bring a Friend.** I have left this one till the end because it is big and controversial, but it doesn't have to be. Remember, this is your relationship and the only two people that make the decisions are you and your partner. Plenty of people do it, and there are many reasons why couples open their relationship up to another person for sexual pleasure.

  This person can be a one-time thing, casually when warranted, or a permanent part of the relationship. Again, your relationship, your choice. This person is, at times, known to the couple, and sometimes a stranger. The most important thing to remember is that all parties involved know the boundaries and communicate thoroughly. There should never be any misunderstandings about what the relationship status is with anyone.

Here are some very important things to consider.

- You need to make sure that your current relationship is solid. If you try to bring in a third party when your relationship is struggling, it won't end well. This is not the type of situation you reach for as a way to save your marriage or relationship.

- If you don't trust each other, this will not work.

- If you don't have a completely honest relationship, this will fail.

- If you are currently having an affair and think by establishing this threesome, you will be free of guilt, think again.

- If you are afraid that your relationship is in jeopardy and if you don't participate, it will end.

These are some important reasons why inviting partners into your relationship will cause significant issues. For this to be successful, it takes planning and open communication. It is also a good move to seek counseling throughout the beginning stages, so boundaries are established, and all of the rules are in place.

Once the person has arrived into your relationship, and all of the boundaries are in place, that is the time to enjoy the newfound freedom and sexual excitement.

Divorce

The dreaded "D" word. There was a time when partners stuck it out no matter the circumstance, but now, we are empowered with resources to try everything we have to work it out, and also make choices to leave if it is in our best interest.

The Excitement

Yes, there are situations when there is a lot of excitement surrounding a divorce. Toxic marriages are filled with narcissistic partners and years of built-up stress, lost sleep, abuse, and trauma. When you find the strength to leave, you have every right to feel excited. Joy for what your future will bring, what new opportunities await, and what freedom may bring for you. Embrace this time, slow down, and take a moment to get to know yourself again.

The Reality

The reality of divorce varies from one person to the next. What we know for sure is that it is a roller coaster of emotions. Here are some realities that everyone should consider.

The end of a relationship or divorce is messy. It affects every area of your life from finances, child custody, your emotions, where you live, and of course, your sex life. When a marriage has broken down so badly that there is no hope for reconciliation, there is an erosion to your union as well as your emotions. There are often acute feelings of bitterness, pain, hatred, shame, embarrassment, fear and even relief all combined in a cacophony of your mind, heart and body. Who's thinking about sex when you're feeling so emotionally raw and drained. I wouldn't be. But in the spirit of holistic health and wellness, it's still important to prioritize your mental and physical wellbeing. Sure, during the messier discussions of splitting your life from your partner and all that involves, it's more important to focus on keeping your head above water and leaning on family, friends and even therapists to support you through. But once the dust has settled on your divorce or breakup, and you've come to the realization that it's time for you to move on without your ex, free yourself from barriers to your happiness.

You are human and sensuality may dim but it never goes away. Dating or having sex with a new partner will be daunting. So start with yourself. Rediscover self-pleasure in your non-marital bed and employ the use of a new sex toy to hit the spot again. It's a major stress reliever. When you're ready to get back out there and meet someone new, for a night, for a season or a lifetime, do your research on what's new on the dating scene and revisit some of the sexual wellness tips and tricks mentioned earlier in this book! You can do it.

The Challenges

The biggest challenge you are going to face during your divorce is balance. How do I balance this new life with my old life? Again, if you have children, that balance will be the forefront of your mind. Being sure all of their needs are being met, having them in family counseling is a great idea. A safe space for them to digest all of their emotions will be helpful for them and you.

Having realistic expectations will also serve you well. Knowing that it is a long process and making sure you have a strong support system in place is vital. Boundaries will also serve you well. Oftentimes, if your partner shares children with you, they will feel they can come and go in your home. Yes, they shared this space with you for a length of time, but those clear lines will help keep things straight for you and the children.

When you are ready to date again, conversations should be had with your children first. Always be sure they understand this is normal, it has no bearing on the relationship you have with them, and never rush a meeting with them and anyone you are dating. This could lead to confusion with children.

Sex After Divorce

The biggest question most ask about sex after divorce is, how long should I wait? Your past relationship possibly left you broken and exhausted. Because of this, you likely are not ready to be intimate with anyone yet.

The number one rule here is, you get to decide when you are ready. This may mean quieting the noise of friends and family who insist all you need is to get back on that horse. Holding on to emotional baggage and bringing that into anyone else's life is not fair to them or you. You deserve the time to heal and if you throw yourself at the first set of genitals that make you tingle, your healing may halt.

The professionals will tell you, if you ignore the fact that you need to heal, you may begin to form some habits that will be toxic to you. What might those habits be? Replacing those feelings with meaningless sex. May seem like a great idea in the beginning, but what typically will happen is once you land in the next committed relationship, if hard feelings show up, you may stray for that meaningless sex to avoid dealing with those feelings.

Now, let's ask the question: Are you going to feel safe and secure during that first sexual encounter? If you were with your partner for a long period of time, this may not have been something you thought about for a long time. The person you were with always knew what you needed.

A brand new human is not going to know you the way your ex did. What you need to feel safe and uninhibited is locked away in your ex-partner's brain. This tells you that you need to be sure you are aware of what you need, and a conversation has to happen before you find yourself naked and unaware of why you feel panicked. You want that first experience after divorce to be wonderful, fulfilling, and pleasurable. To make that happen, give yourself the time needed to ensure it.

On the other hand, some people have been in long and sexless unions and can't wait to put themselves out there and back 'in there'. If you've been sex starved for some amorous congress, have at it. Just be honest with your partner that you have no intention of entering into any serious or longer term relationships and prefer something hot and temporary. We're all in different situations and require different solutions.

I will call this a full circle moment, as we have traveled through dating, long-term relationships, marriage, and divorce. Each of them has their own exciting moments, realities, and challenges. Being aware of them, communicating and being open and honest will help maneuver all of these journeys.

CHAPTER 8: Exciting Your Queer Sexual Connections

"Yes, sex involves our bodies. But it doesn't involve only – or even primarily–our bodies. It's so much more than that"
–Sheila Wray Gregoire

As I discussed earlier in the book, although sex education has come a long way, there are definitely still some major gaps in many school curriculums. Sex ed by and large still focuses on the dangers of sex and not on the full experience of it. Furthermore, the realities of genderqueer individuals are often silenced or unrecognized by most school board programs. Interestingly enough, all youth alike including queer youth are still learning about their sexuality, through self-discovery in spite of the lack of sex education about queer identity.

A GLSEN National School Climate Survey discovered that less than 5% of LGBTQ2S+ students attended a health class that even mentioned a positive LGBTQ2S+ related topic. Self-identified millennials that were surveyed in 2019 stated that only 12% of their sex education classes mentioned same-sex relationships at all (GLSEN, 2015).

As much as I didn't want to have one exclusive chapter just for queer individuals (as I recognize that normalization is key) there are specific considerations that should be highlighted as they have significant impacts on this particular community.

What Is Queer Sex?

Our gender and our sexuality, are all fluid and fluctuating. Queer is a term that speaks to the notion that gender and sexuality are fluid and changing overtime for many. Queer can include transgender, gay, nonbinary, lesbian individuals but there are a lot more identities that can also be included. Likewise, our sexual desire sits on a spectrum much like most parts of ourselves. Queer sex is a broad phrase used to encompass sexual relations between those who do not conform to traditional norms around sexuality and gender or non-heterosexual people or people who don't identify as cisgender or straight.

Defining Trans

Get Real states:

> "Trans refers to individuals who are born or assigned either female or male at birth but whose gender identity does not align or match with that assigned sex (either a little bit or not at all). These include trans men (assigned female at birth and are male identified) and trans women (assigned male at birth and are female identified), and also people who might call themselves any of these very different words: gender queer, gender fluid, ambi gender, and bi gender. And it can also include people who identify as Two-Spirit or Two-Spirited. Indigenous peoples may refer to themselves as being TwoSpirit acknowledging the energy of male

and female spirits they embody. Some trans people express themselves more stereotypically male or female, while others don't. Some trans people opt not to take hormones or have surgery (known as non-op), while others find that medical therapies are necessary for them (known as pre-op or post-op)." (Malone, 2015, p.10)

Dating as a Trans Person

As I've mentioned before, navigating the dating world in the 21st Century can be quite daunting. it's a big world out there and there are many shiny happy faces on dating apps so it can be quite overwhelming. Dating as a trans person is no different and of course has its own specific considerations.

Coming out as trans is a very personal process and decision. There is fear and nervousness of rejection and shame from society, not to mention friends and family. There's also the issue of finances to manage all the potential costs associated with medical and legal requirements when transitioning. For all the emotional, mental, financial and physical impacts this entire process entails a trans person of course wants and deserves to be loved and be desired sexually.

Thankfully there are slowly starting to be more open and safe spaces in communities and online for trans people to network, socialize and meet others. That said, there are still particular challenges that transgendered individuals encounter when dating. Here are a few of the most common:

- **Divulging your identity.** People who identify with the gender they were born with have the privilege of freely expressing who they are especially when it aligns with society's established understanding of masculinity and femininity. As a trans person it can be daunting and scary when dating and especially considering having sex with someone. What is important is to establish a level of trust with your sexual partner before sharing any intimate details of your identity to prevent any unexpected responses. I'll discuss more about this shortly. Ultimately please think about when is the best time to disclose your trans identity whether it be on the first date, on the app or right before you meet.

- **Confidence.** As with everybody else trans persons also need to feel confident when dating and navigating their sexuality. Being naked in front of somebody else can be quite daunting if you're not a supermodel. However for transgender individuals there's also feeling safe when there's a possibility of revealing such items as physical binders and packers during sex. Communication is key to ensure your comfort and trust in your sexual partner before revealing yourself.

- **Sex Drive.** As mentioned earlier for some trans persons, taking hormones will impact your physical body. Some individuals may experience a loss of libido while some individuals may experience an increase in the level of sex drive with a change in your hormone balance. This is a big deal. If you are experiencing a decrease in libido allow time for your body to fully adjust and then taking safe and effective ways to get your mojo back. While on the other hand if with more testosterone you have an increased sex drive, again, take time to settle in this new physical experience and then have at it. It's important to be mindful of the changes occurring in your body, being safe and sexually healthy.

- **Physical changes.** Some trans gendered individuals may choose to undertake a gender reassignment which will include genital surgery. Metoidioplasty and phalloplasty are most common genital surgeries a trans person may have. Like with all surgeries each of these come with their own risk of complications and side effects. It's important for you to allow your body to heal most importantly. For many, genital surgery comes in stages and leads to subsequent surgeries over time. So give yourself time to adjust to a significant change to your body before sharing it with someone else. I suggest you practice with yourself for a little while. Self-pleasure can be a good indicator for how your sexual experiences with someone else will be. So ease into this new sexual experience. It will be better for you and your partner if you are fully comfortable and healthy when it comes to your new body.

Having Sex as a Trans Person

Check in with yourself first. Consent begins by knowing yourself as well as what your boundaries are. Be sure to ask yourself those important questions like what you want out of this sexual experience. Having your own solid boundaries established before bringing in a partner will make this journey that much more enjoyable. Next, you will be ready to have an honest and respectful conversation with your partner. Knowing what they enjoy and what limitations—if they have any—leaves a blank canvas for you both to explore sex toys, creativity, and most of all, pleasure. Here are a few areas you can discuss to make your time together go smoother.

- **Name your naughty parts**. Private parts can get complicated in the queer community. It is safe to say that one of the biggest end goals of sex is for people to feel good in their bodies. You can get a start on this by being upfront about the terms you use for your naughty bits. Be sure to let your partner know how you prefer to be labeled, and ask the important questions. What do they call their bits and how do they like them to be touched?

- **Gender roles can be bendable roles**. The rules that exists between the sheets are the ones you create with your partner. This includes roles. If you prefer to have them, that is fine. Again, the choice is yours. However you identify, that should never determine how you choose to pleasure yourself or someone else.

- **Consent is paramount**. In this pleasurable moment, we want to be sure that consent begins by asking permission prior to any sexual interaction beginning. It is always best to check in as you go, ask if this touch is enjoyable, if that move is pleasurable, and encourage your partner to answer honestly. You would be surprised how many will answer yes to avoid hurting your feelings. We want real feedback here so that pleasure and joy can continue and increase for both partners.

- **Plan your aftercare**. Let's not forget the moments after sex. They can actually be quite awkward. Yes, we all have that, gulp down copious amounts of orange juice, and then remember how hungry we are. But I am talking about aftercare. Have a discussion with your partner about how they like things to be handled after all the joy and pleasure. Do they like to have a shower and head out? Do they want to sleep in? Order sushi? Do you like some quiet alone time and meeting up the next day? We are all different in this approach, but it is worth a conversation. Just be sure that you are both on the same page because nobody likes to be sitting by that phone wondering why they haven't heard from someone after what they thought was an amazing night of connection.

  - **Having Safer Queer Sex.** Hormones are going to come into play here. We are aware that testosterone hormones decrease your risk of unwanted pregnancy, but people on testosterone can still become pregnant. You need to be using condoms because sperm have one job, to swim upstream. Yes, estrogen hormones do indeed slow sperm production, but that makes no difference if you are producing sperm. We know the science, so your egg-dropping partner could find themselves pregnant. Grab that box of condoms before meeting up.

    Hormone therapy can wreak havoc on you. It has been known to fluctuate your sexual libido, and it can make a mess of your emotions. Do yourself a favor and have a strong support system in place for when these times crop up. A counsellor who is sensitive to LGBTQ2S+ lived experiences would be very beneficial. At the very least, keep communicating, because keeping those issues bottled up will do you serious harm.

- **Condoms aren't a one-trick pony.** Condoms significantly reduce pregnancy and STIs for every kind of penetrative sex. They are also great to slide over a sex toy for a quick clean up! When sharing those amazing toys with your partner, you can easily slip that condom off and apply a clean one, and it is safe for them to use.

- **Lube, don't leave home without it.** Lube needs to be mandatory in all sexual encounters. You shouldn't be surprised to hear me say this by now. Water soluble lube works with latex and it drastically reduces friction from both body parts and toys. Get creative and add some lube to the receiver's end of a dental dam. Ever thought of putting a small drop on the inside of a condom *before* you put it on? This makes things a silky, smooth texture for the condom-wearer giving them an increase in pleasure as well. Anal sex also needs lube. Your booty does not self-lubricate like the vagina does, and without the addition of lube, you could end up with painful tearing.

Dating a Trans Person

If you are considering dating a trans person, you may have asked yourself if there are any specific things you should know beforehand. Some may believe that dating is dating is dating. Dating a trans individual is no different to anyone else. That being said, it's important to dig a bit deeper on this to get a clearer idea whether there is truth to this statement.

Dating is always a game of roulette regardless of who you date. You can have an amazing first experience, and the next can be a disaster. This has nothing to do with being a trans individual, this is the world of dating. Nevertheless, dating a trans person may have specific considerations that a non-trans person may be blind to. Raising awareness as a way to demystify and inform will hopefully help reduce discrimination, alienation and even transphobic incidents in society. I have compiled a few considerations for dating transgender women, and then transgender men.

Dating Trans Women

There are some trans woman that have emotional trauma from their past regarding their transition. Be mindful that she may come with some past experiences that were harmful to her. She may have had experiences where she was treated poorly. If you want to be that person who changes that, read on.

- **Don't treat her like a fetish.** Get your fetishes taken care of elsewhere. Keep your inappropriate questions to yourself. Would you be comfortable being asked anything about your genitals before you felt comfortable? Then it would be very inappropriate to ask her if she "tucks her penis." She may not have one at all. If you have a conversation about vaginas, it will never be okay to ask if it looks "real." Does yours? Let's be honest, they all look pretty unique now, don't they? This is an actual real human in front of you, don't be ignorant and treat her as if she has no emotion. It sounds incredible that we're discussing how to treat another person, but apparently these type of questions are all too common.

  I cannot imagine in any world it would be okay to discuss genitals on a first, or even third date if it's not a natural part of the conversation. This goes for dating a trans person as well. All of those personal questions should be saved for when she is ready to have that conversation and not a second before.

- **No awkward compliments please and thank you.** "Man, I was afraid of what you would look like, but you are smoking hot for a trans woman." This is not a compliment. This is a microaggression. Be genuine and sincere by complimenting her laugh, her eyes, or her personality. Trans women have to handle these situations constantly and it is degrading.

- **She didn't transition because of a man**. It is often a mindset that trans women transition so they can have sex with straight men. This is untrue. It is your choice to date her or not. A trans woman can identify as lesbian or bisexual, or want to date a man. She can choose to date whomever she wants.

- **Don't keep her a secret**. If you find yourself attracted to a trans woman and you want to begin a relationship, there should never be a reason you keep her a secret. This is disrespectful, and she deserves better. If you are uncertain or uncomfortable with being in public romantically with someone who is trans, that is your issue. Perhaps you should reconsider being in a relationship with her altogether.

- **Don't expect sex immediately**. Society has often portrayed trans women as sexual fetishes. Please do not expect your date to be this sexual fetish for you. As with non-trans persons, respect her decision if she needs time and space before becoming sexually active. The nature and boundaries of your relationship should be no different from if you were with a non-trans person. If you both are into sexual fetishes or want to engage in casual encounters, have at it. My point is, don't assume sex just because she is a trans woman.

FAQs

Will dating a trans woman change my sexuality?

- One of the first questions many straight people ask before dating a trans person is 'does this make me gay'? The answer is no. You are not gay, and you are not bisexual. If you are attracted to a trans woman, you are attracted to women. A trans woman is a woman. Sexual orientation is not dependent on your attraction to gender. There is a distinction between gender and sex. Sex is fixed and gender is fluid. Spend some time thinking about this for yourself before dating a trans person. Otherwise you might risk mistreating them because you are not fully self-aware and informed.

Dating Trans Men

We have spent time diving into the important considerations for dating a transgender woman, let's now focus on a dating trans men. Similarly to trans women, there may be trans men who have had traumatic experiences attached to their transition. Taking the time to be informed about common lived experiences of trans persons can go a long way to ensuring your partner is treated with respect and dignity. That being said, here are a few considerations for you to think about based on common questions non-trans people have had.

- **Am I gay or straight when dating a trans man**? Dating a trans man does not and will not make you gay unless you are gay. If you identify as a man and are attracted to a trans man, you are gay. If you identify as a woman attracted to a trans man, you are a heterosexual, straight woman. This is the same dynamic as dating non-trans.

- **Will I get the best of both worlds?** A trans man is a man, he is not half-man, half-woman, so no. If you want the best of both worlds, consider being in a polyamorous relationship with both a man and a woman.

- **Can I ask about their surgery**? That's a no. Are you comfortable being asked about your genitals? Please note that not all trans men have surgery. Surgery isn't the end goal for each trans person. From a medical perspective, there is a long waitlist in some countries for gender reassignment surgery. Some transgender men are content to stick with testosterone treatments and some may make a personal choice to stay off them altogether. To avoid any awkward, embarrassing and offensive moments, just employ some sensitivity and discernment. Know that every trans person's journey is different.

- **Don't let sex be scary**. Communication is key here. If you have any issues of nervousness for your first time having sex, have an open and honest conversation before the clothes come off. If you are feeling anxious, you both likely are, it is a new setting and a new person, and this is normal for all partners.

- **Be proud to be with them, or don't be with them at all.** If you have had a conversation about his openness, there should be no reason for you to keep him a secret. If you want to keep it intimate and between friends initially, totally acceptable, but at no point should he feel isolated, alone, or hidden. Transgender men don't need someone in their life who is embarrassed of them. If you can't be supportive and convicted in your decision, please leave them be to find someone who can.

FAQs

What about the lower half?

- You have every right to be informed about the person you are dating. So do your research and get educated prior to broaching the subject with your partner at a reasonable and respectful time. Read your partner's social ques, if he feels uncomfortable about discussing it, drop the subject until he is. Discussing our bodies should be a natural conversation based on interest in getting to know the person we are dating, not for general curiosity.

- To help demystify, generally speaking, when a person who has a vagina begins taking testosterone, their clitoris will grow into a small penis. This is when surgery comes into play, and it will enhance the small clitoris. This surgery is called *metoidioplasty*. Actually, though, the most popular form of genital surgery is called *phalloplasty*. They will remove a portion of your skin from somewhere on your body, called a skin graft, and use it to create a penis.

- Please remember, discussing anyone's genitals before being in a committed relationship is inappropriate. If they choose to share with you sooner, that is their choice. Educating yourself will show support and respect.

Intimate Partner Violence

Intimate partner violence or IPV is unfortunately a too common occurrence in the trans and nonbinary communities. It is an extremely serious issue. According to the National Centre for Transgender Equality (NCTE), "transgender individuals and communities experience shocking amounts of violence and discrimination. In addition to experiencing high rates of domestic and sexual violence, trans and non-binary people are often the targets of transphobic hate crimes and state violence." (National Centre for Transgender Equality, 2016).

The same study found that, "nearly half (46%) of respondents were verbally harassed in the past year because of being transgender, nearly one in ten (9%) respondents were physically attacked in the past year because of being transgender and more than half (54%) experienced some form of intimate partner violence, including acts involving coercive control and physical harm" (National Centre for Transgender Equality, 2016).

The statistics do not change based on the sex assigned at birth. IPV prevalence estimates are comparably high for assigned-male-sex-at-birth and assigned-female-sex-at-birth transgender individuals, and for binary and nonbinary transgender individuals, though more research is needed.

Studies have been done, we know the statistics, and they warrant urgently needed prevention to protect trans and nonbinary people. There continues to be a serious lack of legal protection as well. Transgender people need to be included in the US Preventive Services Task Force recommendations promoting IPV screening in primary care settings. Interventions at the policy level and the interpersonal and individual level are urgently needed to address epidemic levels of IPV in this marginalized, high-risk population (Peitzmeier et al., 2020).

Dating a Nonbinary Person

A nonbinary person will face many societal obstacles when dating as there are so many unspoken expectations based around gender that many don't even realize. Trying to resist societal pressures to fit in a gendered role is oppressive. Not fitting into a heteronormative sexuality may be a significant challenge for those who identify as nonbinary. Nonbinary individuals have been noted to struggle with being misgendered on dating apps as many of them are developed with a gender binary framework in mind. As nonbinary, using more inclusive dating apps that allow you to self-identify would be a less dehumanizing option. There are dating apps such as Lex that operate as a more gender fluid platform.

Similarly to the discussion earlier for trans individuals, nonbinary persons have to be mindful when choosing to disclose their identity when dating. A nonbinary person's sexual attraction doesn't change just because they don't subscribe to a particular gender. This is a key issue. Your sexual preference is based on who you are attracted to just like everyone else. It's also important to know that since so much of what we are all taught about sexuality is based on a concept of masculine and feminine gendered roles. It's a challenge for nonbinary persons to express their own sexuality within these existing sexual paradigms. So when a nonbinary person dates or contemplates having sex with a heterosexual person this may cause that person to question their own sexuality out of ignorance.

Terminology 101

What is nonbinary? It is an identity that does not fit as just male or just female. They identify outside of the masculine or feminine gender binary, hence the term nonbinary. Recently, you might have seen the term "enby" floating around. It is quite commonly used as an abbreviation for nonbinary and is pronounced NB.

You may have already started to be familiar with the more inclusive gender identity language.

- **Cisgender:** You identify with the gender you were assigned at birth.
- **Transgender:** You identify with a gender other than the one they were assigned at birth. You will

also run into circumstances when a transgender identifies as nonbinary.

- **AMAB:** This is an acronym you will hear which translates to assigned male at birth.

- **AFAB:** Another acronym translation to assigned female at birth.

You might be wondering about pronouns and how to use them. When it comes to nonbinary people, they typically follow they, their, them as they are gender neutral. They have been known to also use neo-pronouns and these were created exactly for this reason. A need was spotted for gender-neutral pronouns, so these were created. Xe, ze, and sie would be considered neo-pronouns. If you are wondering what you should be calling your nonbinary person if things become serious, it is best to ask. Most prefer gender-neutral terms like partner or lover to the typical boyfriend and girlfriend, but again, it is best to have that discussion. That said, overtime gender neutral relationship classifications have become normalized regardless of identity.

Who Do Nonbinary People Date?

Just to clarify up front, being nonbinary is about an individual's gender and how they identify as a human. This has no relevance to their sexual orientation. Our gender gives us and others an idea of who we are as a person, while sexual orientation is more indicative of who we are attracted to. When talking about sexuality, the terms don't fit well in the nonbinary world. The terms heterosexual and homosexual automatically assume gender, and therefore, will not work. For this reason, there is a specific vocabulary often used in the nonbinary community when referring to sexuality, of these terms include:

- **Androsexual:** This group identifies as only being interested in males sexually.

- **Gynesexual or Gynosexual:** This group identifies as only being interested in females sexually.

- **Bisexual:** This group identifies as being interested in multiple genders. In the past, this term was used when describing someone interested in two genders, typically only male and female.

- **Pansexual or Allosexual:** This group identifies as being interested in all genders sexually. They don't discriminate between genders.

- **Skiliosexual:** This group identifies as being only attracted to nonbinary people sexually.

- **Asexual:** This group identifies as having next to no sexual attraction. There are occasions when they might still have romantic feelings for someone.

If you're asking yourself, 'How do I know the sexual orientation of a nonbinary person I might want to date?' Well, I would follow up with the question, 'how do you know the sexual orientation of any person you have ever dated?' You probably asked them, right? There's no difference.

Dating tips

Dating in the nonbinary world can present confusion for some, but communication, respect and support are key. Below you will find some useful advice if you are a binary person interested in dating a nonbinary individual.

- **Find out their pronouns**. This will show respect and support from the start. It is also important to use gender-neutral names when introducing your date to others. If you start to get serious, how will you introduce them to your friends and family? What about pet names as your relationship develops?

- **Don't ask about their assigned name**. Many nonbinary persons have been faced with the "before" questions. What was their life like before becoming nonbinary. Yes, we come into this world with a birth name assignment. But consider that if you struggled to identify with that gender assignment at birth, you also couldn't identify with your given name. There may be hurtful memories of confusion related to your given name. It can be traumatizing to relive them, so be considerate and refrain from asking unless your partner brings it up.

- **Ask about introductions**. This might seem so simple to you, but introductions can be a precarious situation for some nonbinary individuals. If they haven't come out to some friends or family because it could be problematic, all it takes is one innocent introduction with a "they" pronoun to set things in motion. Have an immediate conversation about their boundaries and how they want to be introduced in public.

- **They are not teachers**. Being nonbinary, queer, or trans can mean facing questions and having to give explanations about their own personal lives and about the community at large. Many non-queer people want to be allies and genuinely want to learn and be more aware. This is commendable, but at the same time, know that if you are asking questions of a nonbinary person, they have probably gotten the same question, 5 or 10 or 50 times before.

  If you're dating someone who is nonbinary, having to be the teacher and fielding constant questions about them being nonbinary might be the last thing they want out of a dating experience. Instead focus on getting to know them as a unique person on a deeper level. Want to impress them? Do your own research and educate yourself. Be prepared to live in their world by being prepared. It is not their job to educate you on all things nonbinary or queer.

- **Be prepared to be the teacher**. All that being said, it will be your job to educate others in your own life. Once you share or announce to your people that you are dating a nonbinary person, they may have questions. You can choose to answer those you feel are respectful and deserve an answer. To protect your partner from inappropriate questions from your family or friends, let them know they can also educate themselves.

- **Let's just be humans**. Enjoy each other's space. More than anything else, try not to get too caught up in societal labels and expectations. You and your partner can set your own expectations about your relationship, how you interact and what your sexual life will involve. When that time comes, just be in the moment and travel the journey allowing your body to lead the way.

FAQs

Can you date a nonbinary person if you are straight?

- Absolutely, attraction is inclusive, and it doesn't know the boundaries. If you find yourself attracted to a nonbinary person and that is mutual, enjoy.

Is it possible for someone who is nonbinary to also be straight?

- This can be a little on the technical side of things. When we define being "straight" we refer to being attracted to someone of the opposite sex, which puts it all on a binary scale. Nonbinary individuals take themselves off that scale completely. That being said, oftentimes a nonbinary person is exclusively attracted to male or female, so in essence "straight."

If you are interested in a nonbinary person and want to ask them out on a date, what is the best way to do so?

- I would assume that when you ask anyone out, you do so with kindness and respect. The same rules apply here. They are a human with feelings and emotions, those you need to respect. If they reject your offer, remember this has nothing to do with how they identify.

Be mindful that some regular dating rituals like buying flowers or opening car doors may not "fit" within the normal ranges of comfort for some. You can circumvent this by simply opening the channels of communication. You can get the jump on all these awkward moments well in advance just by having an honest conversation.

CHAPTER 9: Harnessing Technology for Sexual Creativity

"Sex times technology equals the future"
—**J.G. Ballard**

Technology has been changing the face of our world for generations. More recently, advancements have been coming faster than ever, and the sexual wellness market is no exception. The big thing we all want to know is, will sextech make our lives better? All the experts agree that this depends on how well we handle the mass influx, both the risks and the benefits.

Sextech covers a wide variety of items. Sex toys, apps, virtual reality, and yes, even sex robots. Most will agree that the new technology can bring positivity to our sexual wellness, a closer connection to both ourselves and our partners. But there are risks involved that we cannot ignore. Privacy and consent are the two biggest things to pay attention to. People want to know if they can get their hands on some of this sextech now, and yes you can, but it will come at a steep price. The experts do expect this market to become more streamlined and therefore, more affordable within the next ten years.

Technology and Sex Toys

There are exciting things coming to the sex toy market. They have spent years studying what the public want and they are ready to deliver. Aiming to fill a void of intimacy and not just sex, you will find robots who can offer an embrace, cuddle or just hold your hand. Recently released in some markets, is a product called "Kissenger" designed to send a kiss long distances. The intent, you place your lips against an artificial mouth, kiss it, and all of the mechanical properties of that kiss are then transferred to your partner's device.

Almost ready for release is a pillow meant to transmit your loved one's heartbeat. Regardless of where you are in the world sleeping, you can still be connected, hearing and feeling their heartbeat. Similarly, already available are completely hands-free toys, used alone or with your partner. To add mystery and intrigue, remote control versions. If your partner is heading off on a business trip, pack that remote in his luggage and he can get you off from the other side of the world. The future is going to the next level with implantation. Some doctors are actively working on electrodes that can be implanted around the spinal code. The idea is that anytime you want that pleasure of an orgasm, you just click a button, and voila. At first glance, most would be adamant that this goes a step too far. In actuality, this could be positive news for those who suffer from certain disabilities that create difficulties with climax.

Will Our Sex Lives Become Virtual

Currently, Virtual Reality or VR technology is expensive. If it becomes more mainstream and in all our homes, sex will most certainly be virtual a lot of the time. In virtual reality, your options are endless. Customize your partner, the activities, and your visual landscape. This is fantasy play at its best. This stretches many people's boundaries, yet many other people are beyond excited about this technology. You can enter a safe space to have mind-blowing sex with a famous person or a deceased spouse. You get to become any person you wish. Remain yourself, or play a fantasy role of your own.

The other amazing benefit of virtual reality for sexual pleasure is how many things you will be able to try that you may have been too shy or afraid to try in actual life. Imagine the possibilities this could afford those who want to safely explore their sexuality. If you want to incorporate your partner, this is another great way to explore fantasies you may have been apprehensive to try before. Sexperts are hopeful that VR will even reduce infidelity because at any time you can jump into the VR world and explore any fantasy you please, without breaking your trust of physical monogamy. There is, most certainly, a chance we move that definition of cheating if this becomes the norm. If your partner feels they are being "replaced" by your VR world, that is a discussion that needs to be had.

Negatives of VR Sex

The biggest concern with VR sex is consent. You having the ability to bring anyone you choose into a virtual world to have sex with them. The debate is, would one be required to obtain consent to have sex with you in a virtual world?

The mental health world has stepped up with some concerns. Those who may struggle with deciphering right from wrong may commit illegal sexual acts in a virtual world. The question being asked is, if they engage in them virtually, will it heighten their need to do it in real life?

When discussing this VR world, most are concerned with the privacy issue first. We all know that what happens online, stays online. In terms of the digital footprint that will be left, who has access to that and what happens if it is leaked, because we all know how easily that can happen.

Lastly, what does this mean for our overall population in the long run? What does the bigger picture look like if most of the population begins to choose virtual sex over real life sex? What does that do to our population? What does this do to our ability to bond and react to one another? Emotions like sympathy and empathy that can only flourish in the company of other humans could become obsolete. Okay, this line of thought maybe becoming a bit conspiracy theory-ish, but you get where I'm going.

Sex Podcasts

Podcasts are all the rage. If you are looking for information on any topic, you can find a podcast on it.

Serious, hilarious, or anywhere in between, you can track down exactly what you desire. The number of sex podcasts available is vast. To make it a bit less overwhelming, you might want to narrow down the topic you want to explore.

Sex podcasts beautifully bring together two things we all want—sex and podcasts—so it makes complete sense that the market is flooded with them. It can be a positive way to get people talking about things that have been taboo for far too long.

These podcasts can discuss topics such as hot sex tips from therapists or the latest and greatest toys on the market. Tune into one that literally dives into each of PornHub's diverse branches. Many say they love these podcasts because they find "their people," a relatable place to laugh, contribute, and even pick up some handy new tricks. Don't hesitate to find one you can tune into with your partner, you both might end up turned on and tuning in every week!

You might get dizzy figuring out where to start, so I have listed a few to get you started.

- **Where Should We Begin with Esther Perel.** This podcast is high on my list of recommendations. She is a relationship therapist, and she invites you into her intimate couple therapy appointments. Visit issues concerning affairs, erectile dysfunction, and sexual concerns. You get an up close and personal look at her suggestions and advice on all sorts of sexual issues. The biggest bonus, you never walk away from an episode without gaining a new and valuable piece of information about sex and relationships.

- **Shameless Sex featuring Amy Baldwin and April Lampert**. This podcast teaches how to feel ultimate pleasure. There are hundreds of podcasts out there filled with information, but this one is the most illustrative. This dynamic duo, Lampert being the sex toy expert, and Baldwin being a sex and relationship coach, they live to show you how to have the best possible sex life. When you tune in you will see refresher courses on masturbation or blowjobs, but don't miss those complex topics. I commend these women for addressing topics most don't touch. Having an amazing sex life when you suffer from chronic pain, how to break into the dominance game or explaining asexuality for everyone to understand.

- **Talk About Gay Sex with Steve Rodriguez.** Steve dishes on all things gay sex. He brings in co-hosts as they dish about funny and personal experiences. Steve covers everything from color changing condoms and douches. Come along for the ride as nothing is off topic, learn about penis size, lube and all the best sex clubs!

Can Reading Erotica Give You Orgasms?

The short answer to that question is yes! The most powerful organ you have in your body is your brain, and with that comes your imagination. Immersing yourself in the world of erotica unlocks all inhibitions and can lead to some amazing orgasms whether you choose to share that time with someone or keep it all to yourself.

A reduced libido and a lack of sexual hunger is the number one complaint women have. They seek out many remedies because they want to feel good; they want pleasure and joy. A recent study has proven that digesting hot, steamy literature can increase your libido and increase the intensity of your orgasm.

The 2016 study, published in the journal *Sexual and Relationship Therapy*, printed the sexual functioning of 27 women over six weeks. 50% of them read self-help books, and 50% read erotic fiction (Palaniappan et al., 2016) Both groups made equal, statistically significant gains when it came to sexual arousal, vaginal lubrication, less pain, satisfaction, orgasms and better sexual experience.

In case you aren't familiar with what erotic literature exactly is, it is typically defined as any type of art that's meant to cause sexual thoughts or arousal (Pietrangelo, 2013). That being said, think pages filled with steamy stories meant to make your toes curl and your juices flow.

The Sex Tape

Mentions of a sex tape can either have someone giddy with excitement or nervous, there is no in between. Many have been made and are floating out there in the cloud. That would explain the uneasiness. When making a consensual sex tape--consensual being the key word there can be invigorating, hot, and heightened pleasure in your bedroom, or wherever you choose to film.

While the good old pornography flicks have been kicking it around here since cavemen were drawing on rocks, sex tapes have only been on the scene since those first grainy, video recorders made it into our hands.

With the invention of the camcorders, we began hearing tales of neighbors and such making the odd tape, but they were still fairly expensive and not many of us had access. Then along came the smartphone and it was sex tape season for all. Yes, people have been taking pictures of their avocado salad and their penises. If you weren't getting the signature dick pic before your first date, was the guy even real?

Why Do We Make Sex Tapes?

Not even the research would be able to predict how many sex tapes are in existence. The bigger question is, why do we make them?

Kayla Lords, sexpert for JackAndJillAdult.com says:

> "Some people want to relive the experience later. They get off on watching themselves (or their partner) experience sexual pleasure. Other people are exhibitionists who want to be watched and making a sex tape can be a great way to do that. And still others (who may also fall into one of the other categories) want to make money from their own amateur porn."(Manley, 2019, para,6.).

Sex Tape Rules

There are most certainly rules involved when dealing with videotaping any type of sexual act. Consent is first on the list. Without consent there is no recording happening, there are severe legal consequences for doing otherwise. Once you and your partner have agreed, talk about boundaries. What are you both comfortable with, who will have possession, and what happens to this file if anything happens to either of you or your relationship? You need to have complete trust in this person. Far too often these cases end up in the hands of legal teams because one angry ex goes rogue, and someone's reputation is forever ruined. You run the risk of your kids, parents, or co-workers finding it. As mentioned, if you don't have full and complete trust in this person, turn the camera off.

Digisexuality

As technology continues to become more intelligent we have started to become more comfortable allowing it to engage in our lives. Just think, where would you be without your phone for a day? Going crazy right? However there are some that have taken their relationships with technology to another level. These individuals have become sexually engaged with computers or should I say robots. Digisexuality, is a term that describes a person's sexual attraction to robots and other forms of technology or artificial intelligence. According to Neil McArthur, 'digisexuality is also emerging as a sexual orientation due to intense sexual and emotional experiences provided by new advances in robotics and artificial intelligence' (McArthur, 2019).

Digisexuality might be confusing to some but the truth is that technology has become integrated in many of our lives. I've spent the past few pages discussing how electronic sex toys, pornography and other technology-based sex products and services have made billions of dollars because apparently, we just can't get enough. Times are changing and technology has become and will continue to become even more integrated into our lives.

CHAPTER 10: Trends in Sexual Wellness

"My tongue can do a better job of teasing you than my words can" –**Unknown**

There is no debate that the sexual wellness market is experiencing an exciting time. More changes are happening than ever before. Innovation and technology are offering us more insight than ever into what our bodies need and what we want. You don't have to look far to find wearable sex technology, extensive and modern period education, and even cyber intimacy. Let's have a closer look at some of the top trends in sexual health and wellness.

As I've discussed earlier, society has started to become more open to recognizing sexual wellness as a part of our holistic wellness. Prioritizing sexual wellness has become a part of a healthy lifestyle. Our thinking around sexuality has also started to expand in progressive ways that hopefully liberate our discomfort from our own human nature. Many of the new sexual wellness trends currently happening are similar to the issues raised earlier in this book.

Lessening stigma. Over the past several years, there has started to be a lessening of the stigma around our bodies – all our bodies and not just of those who are slim. Society is starting to become a lot more body positive and body inclusive in celebrating sexuality. People of all different shapes and sizes are sexy and having sex. There are even more lingerie companies with inclusive sizes and plus sized ad models promoting their brands.

Many grew up with either no discussion regarding masturbation, or were told if they engaged in it, they would go blind or go to hell. I am not joking about this. A part of your own body, that when you touch it, it brings you joy and pleasure. We now have doctors, therapists and adults encouraging self-pleasure to reduce stress, anxiety, and just to help you improve overall health. Seniors are even being encouraged to engage in masturbation as it's great for circulation and mental health.

Women as sexual beings. Women *are* sexual beings! Women have always been but had to be quiet about it because it didn't align with societies expectations. Now more than ever there are sexual wellness products flooding the market that are tailored to vulva owners. I've already shared how explosive the sex toy industry has been, especially for women and female parts. Adult entertainment as a whole has expanded to reach a female market. Books like E.L. James', *Fifty Shades of Grey* took erotic literature mainstream for the first time and made millions doing it. Now there are pornography sites, strip clubs and countless sex shops especially for women.

Gender inclusivity. Society has started to become more gender inclusive with language, policy and education. There is a growing realization that speaking to a particular gender, sex, sexual or pronoun can be limiting and exclusionary to many in society. In an age where diversity and inclusivity has become at the forefront of many discussions, gender inclusivity must be a part of this conversation as well.

Normalizing periods. Most women are capable of menstruating. It's as normal as having sex. Yet women have had to hide periods as something shameful and disgusting. For decades, commercials for menstruation pad brands used blue liquid to show period blood absorption. This is weird because I've never seen blue colored blood. Looks like companies are starting to embrace the reality of periods and are starting to use red liquids. Additionally, many schools in North American and Europe are starting to offer period pads for free in schools, workplaces and other public places recognizing that menstrual products are an essential need.

Menopause education. For generations, women hid the fact that they had a period, then they gave life to children and when they began to age, they had to hide menopause. Most had no idea what was happening and were told they were "going crazy." Hot flashes, mood swings, and feeling miserable was all part of what was expected, and don't dare speak about your symptoms. Now, women are bonding over tricks and tips, and ways to get through it together. Now, women aren't being left in the dark about what their body is going through. They can understand that they can have a healthy sex life by managing the symptoms during this time of their life.

Genital cosmetic surgery. Labiaplasty is the technical term for a vaginal plastic surgery. Between 2013 and 2016, labiaplasty surgeries increased by a whopping 112% (Fight the New Drug, 2019). Many of the candidates for this surgery are young vagina owners who are greatly influenced by watching pornography. Seeing adult film stars with a variety of cosmetic surgeries seem to have an effect on impressionable minds.

Male contraceptive pill. As it stands penis owners can only choose between two effective birth control methods, condoms and a vasectomy. However there has been another form of birth control for men in development. Enter the male birth control pill. There has been ongoing discussion about this contraceptive as it is hormone based and would have to target testosterone. Targeting testosterone would lead to side effects of depression, weight gain, and increased cholesterol levels. Clinical studies to find a contraceptive for males without affecting hormones are on-going.

As we continue to move forward as a society, our ideas and beliefs are changing around sexuality and the trends appearing are reflecting this change. Not every trend or change will be for everyone but more options are exciting and add to the richness of our sexual wellness overall.

Conclusion

What an insightful and educational journey! Beginning with our trip through the early years of sex education, we were able to see exactly where communication around sex all began. This offered us a peek into just how far we have come, with insight into where we need to still improve.

Next, we toured our way into sexual wellness and the importance we need to place on our pleasure, joy, and yes, orgasms. Taking the shame out of sex and making it normal. We traveled the road of sexual health, touching on points of ways to continually improve our wellness. How our physical and emotional health are always front and center and now it is time to bring our sexual health to center stage.

I was excited to hike the hills of sexual pleasure and all of the amazing ways we can incorporate joy, excitement, and yes, those orgasms again into our regular daily life. Bringing to light, tools, and tips shared with you in hopes of sparking some interest that may intrigue or inspire you to treat your whole being to sexual wellness and pleasure.

It was important to trek the precarious paths of mental health and how it plays into your sexual wellness. I hope you refer back to this section often, when you are in need of specific ways to re-center and align your mind, body, and soul.

We wandered the foothills of dating, marriage, and divorce, and how all these different stages impact our sexual wellness. All are unique in their own way and having the knowledge to deal with each of them with support and an open mind can feel empowering.

We sailed our rainbow flag high to assure we covered all things transgender, nonbinary, and queer. Being able to educate and support all communities is vitally important. How to date, explore bodies, and most important, enjoy pleasure and sex.

Carefully traversing the waters of sex tech, this new branch of pleasure is exciting and continues to add things we need to keep an eye out for. Continuously improving ways to please ourselves or our partner, we all need to be excited for the future.

I want to wrap up by thanking you for coming with me on this pleasure journey. Educating and empowering people so there are fewer unknowns, create more pleasurable experiences and make life a lot more exciting. Please refer to the resource section for some fantastic sites on sexual health, safety, and pleasure education. Signing off with wishes of happiness and toe-curling ecstasy.

Resources

This list of resources has been provided to assist you in all things sexual wellness. Resources to help guide you when looking for answers to improve and maintain your sexual wellness.

https://youngwomenshealth.org/

https://youngmenshealthsite.org/

http://www.positive.org/

http://www.itsyoursexlife.com/

http://mysexdoctor.org/

https://www.thetrevorproject.org/

https://rainn.org/

https://pflag.org/

https://www.sexwise.org.uk/

https://www.talktabu.com/

https://afrosexology.com/

https://genderqueer.me/

https://smartsexresource.com/

https://sexpositivefamilies.com/

https://www.sexandu.ca/

https://www.bishuk.com/

https://fumble.org.uk/

https://www.embracesexualwellness.com/

https://getcoral.app/

https://weareferly.com/

https://nishw.org/

https://elnasexualwellness.com/

https://getmaude.com/

https://instituteforsexualwellness.org/

https://nevertmi.ca/

https://www.lover.io/

https://www.brook.org.uk/

https://meetrosy.com/

https://www.wellnessbeyondthebinary.ca/

https://kama.co/

https://www.transwellness.ca/

References

Agnieszka Radzimińska, Agnieszka Strączyńska, Weber-Rajek, M., Styczyńska, H., Katarzyna Strojek, & Zuzanna Piekorz. (2017). *The impact of pelvic floor muscle training on the quality of life of women with urinary incontinence: a systematic literature review*. Clinical Interventions in Aging, 13, 957–965. https://doi.org/10.2147/CIA.S160057

Allan, G. M., & Koppula, S. (2012). *Risks of venous thromboembolism with various hormonal contraceptives*. Canadian Family Physician, 58(10), 1097. https://www.ncbi.nlm.nih.gov/pmc/articles/PMC3470507/

Alptraum, L. (2018, October 28). *The damaging vagina myth we need to stop believing*. Www.refinery29.com. https://www.refinery29.com/en-us/2016/06/113241/porn-pussy-perfect-vagina-myth#slide-1

The American Chemical Society. (2022, March 23). *A non-hormonal pill could soon expand men's birth control options*. American Chemical Society. https://www.acs.org/content/acs/en/pressroom/newsreleases/2022/march/non-hormonal-pill-could-soon-expand-mens-birth-control-options.html

Aquino, L. (2021, July 4). *The beginner's guide to CBD and sex.* Base. https://get-base.com/blog/cbd-sex-benefits

Ashley. (2015, December 7). *12 types of birth control.* Www.plannedparenthood.org. https://www.plannedparenthood.org/planned-parenthood-pacific-southwest/blog/12-types-of-birth-control

Barnes, S. (2021, February 28). *This lesser-known type of sex toy may take your orgasms to the next level.* Mindbodygreen. https://www.mindbodygreen.com/articles/clit-pumping-guide-and-products

Barrosso, A. (2020, August 20). *Key takeaways on Americans' views of and experiences with dating and relationships.* Pew Research Center. https://www.pewresearch.org/fact-tank/2020/08/20/key-takeaways-on-americans-views-of-and-experiences-with-dating-and-relationships/

Bernstein, E. (2021, March 6). *How tech will change sex and intimacy, for better and worse.* Wall Street Journal. https://www.wsj.com/articles/how-tech-will-change-sex-and-intimacy-for-better-and-worse-11615003201

Boom, K. (2022, July 28). *Never experienced A G-spot orgasm? These 9 sex toys will change that.* Mindbodygreen. https://www.mindbodygreen.com/articles/best-g-spot-vibrators

Canadian Mental Health Association. (2021, July 19). *Fast facts about mental health and mental illness.* CMHA National; Canadian Mental Health Association. https://cmha.ca/brochure/fast-facts-about-mental-illness/

CDC. (2019). *Basic statistics.* Centers for Disease Control and Prevention. https://www.cdc.gov/hiv/basics/statistics.html

Centers for Disease Control and Prevention. (2021, January 19). *STD facts - human papillomavirus (HPV).* Centers for Disease Control and Prevention. https://www.cdc.gov/std/hpv/stdfact-hpv.htm

Cohen, S. (2022, March 15). *Suicide rate highest among teens and young adults.* Https://Connect.uclahealth.org/. https://connect.uclahealth.org/2022/03/15/suicide-rate-highest-among-teens-and-young-adults/

Coleridge, S. (2021, February 4). *Work without hope by Samuel Taylor Coleridge.* Poetry Foundation. https://www.poetryfoundation.org/poems/43999/work-without-hope

Collaborative Divorce Texas. (n.d.). *Common sexual problems in marriage.* Collaborative Divorce Texas. Retrieved October 1, 2022, from https://collaborativedivorcetexas.com/common-sexual-problems-marriage/

Daniela. (202 C.E., March 24). *Hot and sexy dirty talk that will spice up your love life.* Www.lovearoundme.com.

https://www.lovearoundme.com/blog/hot-and-sexy-dirty-talk-that-will-spice-up-your-love-life.html

Data Bridge Market Research. (2022, July 15). *Sexual wellness market to portray USD 17.14 billion, with growing CAGR of 6.57% during forecast period 2022 to 2029 | analyzed by size, share, growth, trends and recent developments. GlobeNewswire NewsRoom.* https://www.globenewswire.com/en/news-release/2022/07/15/2480207/0/en/

Davidson, K. W., Barry, M. J., Mangione, C. M., Cabana, M., Caughey, A. B., Davis, E. M., Donahue, K. E., Doubeni, C. A., Krist, A. H., Kubik, M., Li, L., Ogedegbe, G., Pbert, L., Silverstein, M., Simon, M. A., Stevermer, J., Tseng, C.-W., & Wong, J. B. (2021). *Screening for chlamydia and gonorrhea.* JAMA, 326(10), 949. https://doi.org/10.1001/jama.2021.14081

Dean, E. (2022, July 18). *Communication strategies for couples seeking third person | regain.* Www.regain.us. https://www.regain.us/advice/marriage/communication-strategies-for-couples-seeking-third-person/

Drouin, M., Coupe, M., & Temple, J. R. (2017). *Is sexting good for your relationship*? It depends …. Computers in Human Behavior, 75(C), 749–756. https://doi.org/10.1016/j.chb.2017.06.018

The Editors. (2022, March 1). *61 sex games that'll spice up any relationship. Cosmopolitan.*

https://www.cosmopolitan.com/sex-love/g3801/naughty-sex-games/

Engle, G. (2020, February 7). *How to give someone the best damn oral sex of their life.* Www.refinery29.com. https://www.refinery29.com/en-ca/how-to-give-best-oral-sex

Ford, T., McCharen, B., & Sicardi, A. (2016, March 11). *Gen Z goes beyond gender binaries in new innovation group data.* Wunderman Thompson. https://www.wundermanthompson.com/insight/gen-z-goes-beyond-gender-binaries-in-new-innovation-group-data

Fight The New Drug. (2019, August 28). *Porn is inspiring teen girls to undergo this invasive and painful cosmetic surgery.* Fight the New Drug. https://fightthenewdrug.org/growing-trend-of-porn-inspired-plastic-surgery-for-teens/

Frank, S. (2020). *Queering menstruation: Trans and nonbinary identity and body politics.* Research Gate. https://doi.org/10.111/soin.12355

Ford, J. S., Shevchyk, I., Yoon, J., Chechi, T., Voong, S., Tran, N., & May, L. (2022). *Risk factors for syphilis at a large urban emergency department.* Sexually Transmitted Diseases, 49(2), 105–110. https://doi.org/10.1097/OLQ.0000000000001543

Ford, T., McCharen, B., & Sicardi, A. (2016, March 11). *Gen Z goes beyond gender binaries in new innovation group data.* Wunderman Thompson.

https://www.wundermanthompson.com/insight/gen-z-goes-beyond-gender-binaries-in-new-innovation-group-data

Gainsburg, M., Blades, N., & Siclait, A. (2021, October 13). *Tonight's the night to try the seated wheelbarrow sex position.* Women's Health. https://www.womenshealthmag.com/sex-and-love/a19943165/sex-positions-guide/

Garcia, J. R., Lloyd, E. A., Wallen, K., & Fisher, H. E. (2014). *Variation in orgasm occurrence by sexual orientation in a sample of U.S. singles.* The Journal of Sexual Medicine, 11(11), 2645–2652. https://doi.org/10.1111/jsm.12669

Gilbert, L. (2020). *Hey, You Got This: Hey, Let's Talk About Sexual Wellness on Apple Podcasts.* Apple Podcasts. https://podcasts.apple.com/us/podcast/hey-lets-talk-about-sexual-wellness/id1503583340?i=1000486504216

Gillen, M. M., & Markey, C. H. (2018). *A review of research linking body image and sexual well-being.* Body Image, 31, 191–197. https://doi.org/10.1016/j.bodyim.2018.12.004

GLSEN. (2015). *Lack of comprehensive sex education putting LGBTQ youth at risk*: National O. GLSEN. https://www.glsen.org/news/lack-of-sex-education-putting-lgbtq-youth-risk

Gracia, Z. (2022, March 11). *What is sexual wellness and why does it matter?* BetterMe Blog. https://betterme.world/articles/sexual-wellness/

Green, A. (2021, June 8). *How to mix sex with food for the best foreplay ever.* YourTango. https://www.yourtango.com/2013181036/food-foreplay-101-7-tips-using-food-bedroom

Grey, J. (2022, March 30). *Body parts aren't gendered. so why are sex toys?* Wired. https://www.wired.com/story/sex-toy-gender-rant/

Hamilton, J. (2020, November 19). *How to use your brain to have better sex.* Oprah Daily. https://www.oprahdaily.com/life/relationships-love/a34483512/mindful-sex/

Harvard Health Publishing. (2022). *Can supplements save your sex life?* Harvard Health. https://www.health.harvard.edu/staying-healthy/can-supplements-save-your-sex-life

Haynes, M. (2008). Re: Thomas LC, et al. *Premanipulative testing and the velocimeter.* Manual Therapy (2007), doi:10:1016/j.math.2006.11.003. Manual Therapy, 13(1), e4. https://doi.org/10.1016/j.math.2007.09.008

Healthline. (2018, May 21). *Female sex hormones: Types, effect on arousal, and 8 other functions.* Healthline. https://www.healthline.com/health/female-sex-hormones#after-childbirth-and-breastfeeding

Hot Blue. (2015, May 15). *Urban Dictionary: palm job.* Urban Dictionary.

https://www.urbandictionary.com/define.php?term=palm%20job

Howard, M. (2021, October 15). *Try one of these moves with your S.O. if your sex life is in a rut.* Women's Health. https://www.womenshealthmag.com/sex-and-love/a19964722/spice-up-sex-life-with-kink

Healthline. (2018, May 21). *Female sex hormones: Types, effect on arousal, and 8 other functions.* Healthline. https://www.healthline.com/health/female-sex-hormones#after-childbirth-and-breastfeeding

Hirschman, C. (2018, June 27). *What is an intimacy coach?* SexCoaching.com. https://www.sexcoaching.com/types-of-therapy/what-is-an-intimacy-coach/

Hsieh, C. (2017, July 11). *13 ways to use lube during sex.* Cosmopolitan; Cosmopolitan. https://www.cosmopolitan.com/sex-love/advice/a226/lube-during-sex/

Hsieh, C., & Varina, R. (2021, December 20). *Everything you ever wanted to know about nipple clamps, right this way.* Cosmopolitan. https://www.cosmopolitan.com/sex-love/a21525813/how-use-nipple-clamps/

Hutchings, A. B. last updated C. from E. (2022, August 3). *What is tantric sex?* How to enjoy tantric sex with your partner. GoodTo. https://www.goodto.com/wellbeing/relationships/tantric-sex-69302

Johnson, M. (2019, March 8). *Is outercourse a real thing?* Healthline. https://www.healthline.com/health/healthy-sex/outercourse#takeaway

Jenkins, W. (2020). *The sensible sexpert.* The Sensible Sexpert. https://www.thesensiblesexpert.com/about

Kappler, M. (2021, November 22). *Why a potentially illegal form of sex therapy has so many defenders.* Healthing.ca. https://www.healthing.ca/wellness/sex/sexological-bodywork#:~:text=It

Kassel, G. (2022, March 28). *7 of the best double-ended dildos for doubling pleasure in solo and partnered play.* Well+Good. https://www.wellandgood.com/best-double-ended-dildos/

Kassel, G., & Miller, K. (2022, July 18). *The 25 best strap-ons to take your sex life to the next level.* Women's Health. https://www.womenshealthmag.com/sex-and-love/g35229125/best-strap-ons/

Keller, A. (n.d.). *Sleep apnea and sex: 4 facts you should know.* WebMD. Retrieved September 13, 2022, from https://www.webmd.com/connect-to-care/sleep-apnea/facts-about-sleep-apnea-and-sex#:~:text=Sleep%20apnea%20can%20decrease%20your%20sex%20drive.&text=The%20study%20also%20found%20a

Lastella, M., O'Mullan, C., Paterson, J. L., & Reynolds, A. C. (2019). *Sex and sleep: Perceptions of sex as a sleep promoting behavior in the general adult population.* Frontiers in Public Health, 7. https://doi.org/10.3389/fpubh.2019.00033

Lee, S. (2020). *Breast cancer statistics.* Canadian Cancer Society. https://cancer.ca/en/cancer-information/cancer-types/breast/statistics

Liao, P., & Dollin, J. (2012). *Half a century of the oral contraceptive pill historical review and view to the future.* Reflections, 58, 757–760. https://www.cfp.ca/content/cfp/58/12/e757.full.pdf

Malone, R. (2015). *Get real a question and answer guide for dating trans folks.* In Get Real (p. 10). Rainbow Health Ontario. https://rainbowresourcecentre.org/files/GetReal-RRC.pdf

Mandriota, M. (2022, May 27). *Experts say these are the top 10 sexual wellness trends to watch.* Psych Central. https://psychcentral.com/sex/top-10-sexual-health-and-wellness-trends-2022#looking-ahead

Manley, A. (2019, December 18). *Shooting your own porn is tricky — here's how to do it right.* AskMen. https://ca.askmen.com/top_10/dating/7-smartphone-sex-tape-tips.html

Markets, R. and. (2021, October 15). *Global sexual wellness market (2021 to 2026) - featuring diamond products, reckitt benckiser and okamoto industries among others.* GlobeNewswire News Room. https://www.globenewswire.com/news-release/2021/10/15/2314887/28124/en/Global-Sexual-Wellness-Market-2021-to-2026-Featuring-Diamond-Products-Reckitt-Benckiser-and-Okamoto-Industries-Among-Others.html

Mark Manson. (2014, January 23). *A Brief History of Male/Female Relations.* Mark Manson. https://markmanson.net/male-female-relations

Mayo Clinic. (2022, September 22). *Kegel exercises: A how-to guide for women.* Mayo Clinic. https://www.mayoclinic.org/healthy-lifestyle/womens-health/in-depth/kegel-exercises/art-20045283

McArthur, Neil & Twist, Markie L.C. (2017) *The rise of digisexuality: therapeutic challenges and possibilities.* Journal of Sexual and Relationship Therapy.

McIntosh, J. (2018, November 23). *Orgasms: Facts, types, causes, and misconceptions.* Www.medicalnewstoday.com. https://www.medicalnewstoday.com/articles/232318#what-is-an-orgasm

Meyerowitz, A. (2020, February 25). *Want to excite your partner? This is what you need to dress up as in bed.* Red Online. https://www.redonline.co.uk/health-self/relationships/a31091614/popular-bedroom-role-play-survey/

Miller, K., & Gainsburg, M. (2022, May 20). *11 best sex pillows*. Women's Health. https://www.womenshealthmag.com/sex-and-love/a20682700/sex-pillow/

Muise, Amy and Impett, Emily A. 'Good, Giving, and Game: The Relationship Benefits of Communal Sexual Motivation', Social Psychological and Personality Science. Volume 6, Issue 2. October 10, 2014. https://doi.org/10.1177/194855061455364

Muise, Amy , 'Are You GGG? Understanding the benefits of sexual communal strength'. Psychology Today. August 12, 2012. https://www.psychologytoday.com/ca/blog/the-passion-paradox/201208/are-you-ggg

Nast, C. (2015, April 1). 15 Shower Sex Positions and Steamy Tips to Try Tonight. Glamour. https://www.glamour.com/story/4-sex-positions-that-are-perfe

Nast, C. (2016, July 20). *21 foreplay ideas & tips you'll be dying to try*. Glamour. https://www.glamour.com/story/new-foreplay-ideas

Nast, C. (2019a, February 14). *What it's like to date when you're nonbinary*. Teen Vogue. https://www.teenvogue.com/story/what-dating-and-love-is-like-for-10-non-binary-people

Nast, C. (2019, June 13). *7 Podcasts That Will Make You Better in Bed*. GQ. https://www.gq.com/story/best-sex-podcasts

Nast, C. (2021a, January 28). *3 reasons to start a sex journal—and how to do it.* SELF. https://www.self.com/story/sex-journal

Nast, C. (2021, June 25). *16 suction vibrators that give your clit all the attention it deserves.* Glamour. https://www.glamour.com/gallery/best-suction-toys

Nast, C. (2022, August 8). *The best cock rings for harder hard-ons.* GQ. https://www.gq.com/story/best-cock-ring

National Center for Transgender Equality (NCTE), 2015 "U.S. Transgender Survey Report"(2016),https://vawnet.org/publisher/national-center-transgender-equality-ncte

Olsen, B. (2021, March 3). *10 ways to navigate dating as a non-binary person.* LGBTQ and ALL. https://www.lgbtqandall.com/*10-ways-to-navigate-dating-as-a-non-binary-person/*

O'Mann, J. (2021, August 17). *Personal hygiene challenges for nonbinary people.* OutCare. https://www.outcarehealth.org/personal-hygiene-challenges-for-nonbinary-people/

Palaniappan, M., Mintz, L., & Heatherly, R. (2016). *Bibliotherapy interventions for female low sexual desire: Erotic fiction versus self-help.* Sexual and Relationship Therapy, 31(3), 1–15. https://doi.org/10.1080/14681994.2016.1158805

Peach, Katherine. 'What Does GGG Mean and Does It Work'? O.School.

https://www.o.school/article/what-does-ggg-mean. September 24, 2021.

Peitzmeier, S. M., Malik, M., Kattari, S. K., Marrow, E., Stephenson, R., Agénor, M., & Reisner, S. L. (2020). *Intimate Partner Violence in Transgender Populations: Systematic Review and Meta-analysis of Prevalence and Correlates. American Journal of Public Health*, 110(9), e1–e14. https://doi.org/10.2105/ajph.2020.305774

Pietrangelo, A. (2013, July 5). *What are sexual norms?* Healthline; Healthline Media. https://www.healthline.com/health/what-are-sexual-norms

The Power to Decide. (n.d.). *Find your birth control method 2020 | power to decide.* Powertodecide.org. Retrieved September 29, 2022, from https://powertodecide.org/sexual-health/your-sexual-health/find-your-method

Proschan, K. (2021, May 6). *Microdosing hormones expands gender-affirming care options for non-binary folks.* San Francisco AIDS Foundation. https://www.sfaf.org/collections/beta/microdosing-hormones-expands-gender-affirming-care-options-for-non-binary-folks/

Public Health England. (2018, June 26). *Survey reveals women experience severe reproductive health issues.* GOV.UK. https://www.gov.uk/government/news/survey-reveals-women-experience-severe-reproductive-health-issues

Queer In the World. (2021, September 16). *What you need to know before dating a transgender person!* Explained. https://queerintheworld.com/dating-a-transgender-person/

Raman, R. (2022, June 10). *7 foods and supplements to boost your libido.* Healthline. https://www.healthline.com/nutrition/viagra-foods#maca

Reason, K. (2022, July 25). *Why and how you should use mirrors during sex.* Love Hope Adventure. https://lovehopeadventure.com/why-mirrors-are-great-to-use/

Redbook. (2018, March 16). *These oral sex tips will blow him away in bed.* Redbook. https://www.redbookmag.com/love-sex/sex/advice/g696/oral-sex-tips/

Reaver, A. (2019, April 10). *How Do Our Sex Hormones Change As We Age?* Blog.insidetracker.com. https://blog.insidetracker.com/changing-sex-hormones

Rider, J. R., Wilson, K. M., Sinnott, J. A., Kelly, R. S., Mucci, L. A., & Giovannucci, E. L. (2016). *Ejaculation frequency and risk of prostate cancer: Updated results with an additional decade of follow-up.* European Urology, 70(6), 974–982. https://doi.org/10.1016/j.eururo.2016.03.027

Roser, M., Ortiz-Ospina, E., & Ritchie, H. (2013). *World population growth. Our world in data.*

https://ourworldindata.org/world-population-growth

Rowland, D., & Gutierrez, B. (2017). *Phases of the human response cycle.* The SAGE Encyclopedia of Abnormal and Clinical Psychology, 62, 1705–1706. https://doi.org/10.4135/9781483365817.n684

Santos-Longhurst, A. (2019, February 27). *Why bother with dry humping?* Healthline. https://www.healthline.com/health/healthy-sex/dry-humping#with-a-partner

Sethi, S. (2021, February 28). *Touch & pleasure are essential: Here's how to give them to yourself : Life kit.* NPR.org. https://www.npr.org/2021/02/16/968355814/touch-pleasure-are-essential-heres-how-to-give-them-to-yourself

Sexual-Wellness-Market-to-Portray-USD-17-14-Billion-with-Growing-CAGR-of-6-57-During-Forecast-Period-2022-to-2029-Analyzed-by-Size-Share-Growth-Trends-and-Recent-Developments.html

Smith, J. (2018, March 1). *Oral contraceptives (birth control pills) and cancer risk - national cancer institute.* Www.cancer.gov. https://www.cancer.gov/about-cancer/causes-prevention/risk/hormones/oral-contraceptives-fact-sheet#r9

Sommer, PhD, R. (2022, September 17). *How to use anal toys, according to A sex educator.* My Sex Toy

Guide. https://www.mysextoyguide.com/how-to-use-anal-toys/

Srikanth, A. (2021, June 23). *Groundbreaking study reveals how many nonbinary Americans there are right now.* The Hill. https://thehill.com/changing-america/respect/diversity-inclusion/559875-groundbreaking-study-reveals-how-many-non-binary/

Staff, D. (2021, April 26). *6 divorce realities you need to know before deciding to divorce.* Divorced Moms. https://divorcedmoms.com/6-divorce-realities-you-need-to-know-before-deciding-to-divorce

Steinburg, Dr. (2019, May 24). *Sex therapy : Options to restore natural sexual health in Montreal.* ELNA Sexual Wellness. https://elnasexualwellness.com/what-is-sex-therapy-anyway/#:~:text=By%20understanding%20and%20dismantling%20old

Stewart, L. (2021, June 10). *How many couples REALLY have sex on their wedding night?* Wedding Journal. https://www.weddingjournalonline.com/how-many-couples-really-have-sex-on-their-wedding-night/#:~:text=We%20carried%20out%20our%20(not

Stubbs, M. (2021). *Playing without a partner.* In www.simonandschuster.com. Cleis Press. https://www.simonandschuster.com/books/Playi

ng-Without-a-Partner/Megan-Stubbs/9781627783040

Sullivan, C., & Hsieh, C. (2022, August 22). *These beginner-friendly BDSM toys will help ya dip your toes into the world of kink.* Cosmopolitan. https://www.cosmopolitan.com/sex-love/advice/g2550/light-bondage-sex-toys/

Sylver, L. (2022, January 22). *Everything you need to know about rimming.* Promescent Better in Bed. https://www.promescent.com/blogs/learn/rimming

Tallon-Hicks, Y. (2019, June 4). *Queer sex 101: How to have sex and do it safely.* Teen Vogue. https://www.teenvogue.com/story/how-to-have-queer-sex

Team, M. (2020, August 11). *A brief history of the condom.* Maude. https://getmaude.com/blogs/themaudern/a-brief-history-of-the-condom#:~:text=In%201839%2C%20inventor%20Charles%20Goodyear

Team, T. L. (2021, November 17). *Body positivity: Having sex with confidence.* Lover App Inc. https://www.lover.io/post/body-positivity#:~:text=What

Tempera, J., & Siclait, A. (2022, April 19). *Wax play might be the perfect kinda-kinky act your sex life is missing.* Women's Health. https://www.womenshealthmag.com/sex-and-love/a29785476/wax-play/

Vered Counseling. (2019, April 3). *How can I deal with gender dysphoria?* Vered Counseling | Kimberly Vered Shashoua, LCSW. https://www.veredcounseling.com/blog/2019/3/26/how-can-i-deal-with-gender-dysphoria

Walansky, A., & Felman, A. (2020, June 29). *The experts taught us how to go down on women correctly.* Greatist. https://greatist.com/live/cunnilingus-tips#gentle-pressure-on-the-pelvis

Wattie, A. (2020, January 11). *What is somatic sex education?* - dame. Dame.com. https://dame.com/what-is-somatic-sex-education/

Young, S. (2017, July 3). *Girls "as young as nine" are seeking vagina surgery because of porn.* The Independent. https://www.independent.co.uk/life-style/gynaecology-girls-aged-nine-vaginal-cosmetic-surgery-pornography-social-media-naomi-crouch-paquita-de-zulueta-a7821186.html

Zane, Z. (2021, January 21). *The 12 best sexy handcuffs and restraints for some BDSM action.* Men's Health. https://www.menshealth.com/sex-women/g35267582/best-sex-handcuffs-restraints/

Zindzi Gracia. (2022, March 11). *What is sexual wellness and why does it matter?* BetterMe Blog. https://betterme.world/articles/sexual-wellness/

www.ingramcontent.com/pod-product-compliance
Lightning Source LLC
Chambersburg PA
CBHW070400120526
44590CB00014B/1190